KNOW MORE

WEIGH LESS

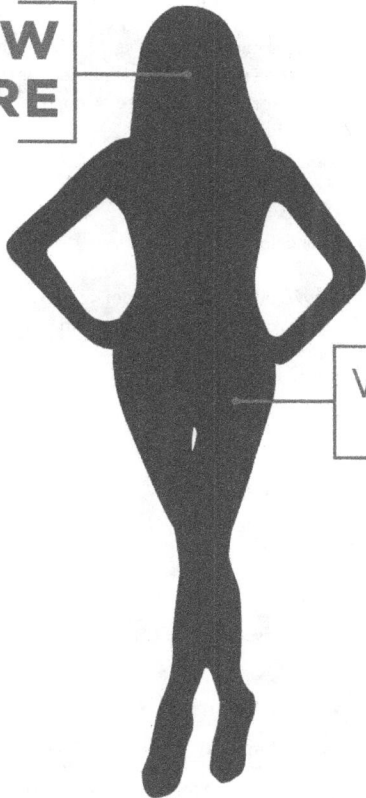

Dr. O's Guide to Scale Bliss

• TINUADE OLUSEGUN, MD •

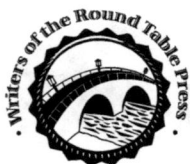

Round Table Companies
1670 Valencia Way
Mundelein, IL 60060

www.roundtablepress.com
www.roundtablecompanies.com

The Writers of the Round Table Press name and logo are trademarks of Round Table Companies.

Publisher: Corey Michael Blake
Executive Editor: Katie Gutierrez Painter
Editor: Kristin Westberg
Production Manager: Erin Cohen
Digital Distribution: David C. Cohen
Cover Design: Analee Paz
Interior Design/Layout, Back Cover: Sunny DiMartino
Proofreading: Rita Hess
Last Looks: Mary Laine

Printed in the United States of America

ISBN: 9781610660433

First Edition: December 2011
10 9 8 7 6 5 4 3 2 1

*A huge thank you to my heavenly father for
making this possible. For without Him I can
do nothing; but with Him all things are possible.*

*And to my family, thank you all for being
there for me through "thick and thin."*

"As a former colleague of Dr. O's and a physician who has been in a similar position with her own patients, I read with great interest the introduction to *Know More, Weigh Less*. I have always admired Dr. O for her tenacity, her dedication to the practice of medicine, and her passion for understanding the workings of the human body. I am certain that her book will reflect these qualities. That Dr. O developed these strategies based on her own personal experiences leaves no doubt in mind that they will be successful for others."

—**Jasmine K. Sawhney, MD**
Child, Adolescent & Adult Psychiatrist

CONTENTS

PART II: WHAT ARE MY OPTIONS?

INTRODUCTION

EAT LESS, EXERCISE MORE.

That's a mantra you've probably been hearing for years, maybe even all your life. In countless variations, you've heard it from family, friends, and colleagues, from the media, from your doctor, and everyone in between. As a physician, it's advice I've doled out dozens of times to overweight and obese patients. And when I gained weight, it's what I told myself.

As a child and teenager in Nigeria, and then a young adult in the U.S., I was never considered overweight. I stood almost six feet tall and weighed about 180 pounds, placing my BMI around 24—normal range. Then life happened. In my late twenties, a serious relationship ended, and I dropped every good habit I'd formed around healthy eating and working out. I ate everything I knew was bad for me and didn't care. My bike grew a layer of dust, and my gym membership expired. By the time I realized how depressed I was, it was too late: I had gained 25 pounds through emotional eating, pushing my weight to 205. I eventually got married, but the weight kept climbing. I gained even more while trying to balance the stress of my medical residency training, married life, and pregnancy. Those first 25 pounds soon became over 50 pounds. By the time my son was born, I weighed in at over 230 pounds. My BMI was now well in the obese category (at around 32), and I knew something had to change.

Step 1: Eat less.

I read every food label to make sure I was not consuming too many calories, too many carbs, too much fat, too much sodium, too much anything. I avoided artificial sugars. I did not drink sodas. And I tried every kind of diet—Atkins, South Beach, Mediterranean—all the popular ones that people have claimed success on and then some of my own (ahem, oatmeal). I was not successful on any of them. The hunger, the lack of energy, the cravings, and the limitations on what I could and could not eat made it difficult to stick with anything long enough to see significant results. I dreaded my boring, low-cal meals, and—except for a few pounds here and there—the weight I needed and wanted to shed wouldn't disappear.

Step 2: Exercise more.

When I realized my diets were failing me, I increased the intensity of my workouts. I rode my bike several miles to the gym, exercised for an hour, and then rode back home. Every day I repeated this routine. I was building some muscle, but for all the sweat and effort I was putting in, the eight pounds I lost over a course of *months* were not enough for me. So I hired a personal trainer and lost another eight pounds. Unfortunately, the vigorous workouts soon took a toll on my Achilles tendon and knees, and I was forced to reduce the intensity after consulting with an orthopedic doctor for my musculoskeletal problems. Inevitably, those few pounds I had worked so hard to lose crept right back on.

Before I fought obesity myself, I viewed it as a disorder in which a person has accumulated excess fat from overeating or not exercising enough. I inwardly rolled my eyes when patients insisted, "Doctor, I'm trying!" I thought, *Yeah, right!* But after experiencing firsthand the frustration of eating less, exercising more, and seeing *no* results, I realized that the weight loss journey is not an easy one. It can be a lonely and isolating road, and I grew determined to find a better solution to losing weight than what we had been telling our patients. That was when my quest began.

My first task was to gain a better understanding of obesity. I put all my research skills to use and read through endless amounts of medical and popular literature. I sorted through the many schools of thought on this disease and looked into dozens of diet and exercise routines, as well as alternative solutions. Finally, I concluded that, when it comes to obesity, one size does *not* fit all.

Contrary to popular belief, obesity is a mysterious disease, and its true definition and actual etiology is highly debated. So many factors contribute to weight gain that I do not believe you can chalk it up to one cause alone. Indeed, with so many different schools of thought, the true answer probably lies somewhere in between. What does this mean for you, for me, for anyone fighting obesity?

It means that even if we can't quite define it, we also can't ignore it. The health risks and conditions that come with obesity are real, and they are life threatening. The situation is too serious to continue serving out the same tired advice: eat less, exercise more. It's not that simple. My hope is that this book will help you discover how *you*—not your sister, neighbor, colleague, or friend— gained the weight ... and what will help *you* lose it for good. I know this journey has been long and difficult. I've walked the same road. And that's why I am here today.

—Dr. O

PART I

WHAT IS OBESITY?

CHAPTER I

THE MYSTERIOUS
DISEASE

READY FOR A KICK IN THE GUT?

Here goes: obesity is one of the leading causes of preventable deaths worldwide, especially in developed nations. In the U.S., it is currently #2 and soon to surpass smoking as #1. In technologically advanced nations, the obesity rate has doubled since the 1980s. Doubled! In the U.S., in particular, almost 60 percent of people fall into either the overweight or obese category. So, if one-third of adults are obese and one-third of adults are overweight, at least one out of every three people you know has a problem with this disorder. In fact, the World Health Organization believes that obesity is one of this century's biggest and most serious public health concerns.

Obesity is our bubonic plague.

So what are we doing about it? Millions of dollars are being spent every year as we work to better understand the signaling pathways and complex areas associated with the obesity epidemic. Some research findings have been promising, but there's still a lot for us to learn.

What we do know is that where you live in the U.S. can affect your weight. In the South, 30 percent of people are overweight or obese; in the Midwest, 28 percent; the Northeast, 25 percent; and about 24 percent of individuals living in the West struggle with their waistlines. The culture, lifestyle, and types of foods people consume in specific areas have huge impacts on these numbers.

Obesity rates also vary by ethnic groups. An article in a well-known medical journal called *JAMA* found up to 44 percent of non-Hispanic blacks are obese; 39 percent of Mexican-Americans; 37 percent of all Hispanics; and around 32 percent of non-Hispanic whites. In total, somewhere between 30 and 40 percent of Americans are considered obese.

Another fact? It's *expensive* to be obese. Whether you're paying to try to lose the weight or spending money on medical bills due to related conditions, you are spending more than your normal-weight counterpart. This is particularly problematic considering the Centers for Disease Control (CDC) study showing that lower income and less-educated individuals, especially women, are more likely to be obese, compared to their higher-earning counterparts.

Even scarier, the number of *children* being classified as overweight and obese has tripled and continues to grow, with 15 percent of children in the U.S. currently falling into that category. Overweight children have increased chances of becoming obese adults and suffering disabilities and premature death, so there's an urgent push to make kids more active and to teach them better eating habits at an earlier age. An example of one such initiative is Michelle Obama's "Let's Move!" campaign (www. letsmove.gov), which aims to put healthier foods in schools and encourage more physical education and activities. Initiatives such as this are invaluable, because they go past statistics to start creating *solutions*.

Still, all of this begs an obvious question: what's causing obesity?

DEFINING OBESITY

What is obesity? This seems like an easy question to answer; I mean, we all know it when we see it, right?

According to the dictionary, obesity is "a condition characterized by the excessive accumulation and storage of fat in the body." Other definitions, including medical ones, might add that obesity can lead to adverse health effects and decreased life expectancy. The CDC mentions that obesity is categorized based on Body Mass Index (BMI), which is an index-based number reached by combining an individual's weight and height.

Okay ... but what factors (besides food) lead to that excessive accumulation and storage of fat? In comparable situations, what makes one person fat where another stays thin? And once the fat builds, why is it so hard to lose? Why, when I ate less and exercised more, could I not drop the weight?

One problem is that the current definition of obesity is too limited. We give a crayon drawing explanation of what the disease looks like once it's already set in but provide no detail, no insight, as to its origin. Why is this? After all, we do such a good job of explaining other medical conditions.

We define them thoroughly and explain their causes, often down to the cellular level, as well as prognoses and treatment options. For example, when a patient comes into my office with diabetes, I can say, "You're not metabolizing sugar properly because you're either not secreting enough insulin or your body has become resistant to that insulin." I can say, "Here's what we think causes this problem, and here's what you can do about it."

Not so with obesity. It's more complicated than that. And, believe it or not, I can't look patients in the eye and say, "Your disease is that you have too much body fat." Can you imagine the stares? That's like saying, "You can't see because you're blind." Well, obviously. "But what caused the blindness?" a patient might ask. "And what can I do to regain my sight?" Not having answers to those questions wouldn't be acceptable, and not having answers for my patients with obesity is not acceptable to me.

THE FAT CELL

So what do we know about obesity so far? It's a complex disease with a problematically simple definition. In order to start learning more, we need to get back to basics: the fat cell.

The nature of the fat cell is very interesting. We should all have a limited amount of fat cells, the first set of which is developed during the third trimester of our mothers' pregnancies. The next time we produce fat cells is during puberty. At this time, the sex hormones of estrogen and testosterone trigger signals in the body to start making fat cells so that we can differentiate what we call "girls" or "boys" from "women" or "men." Women will develop fat cells in their breasts, hips, and waists; and men will produce them in their chests, abdomens, and buttocks. Theoretically, these two times in our lives are the *only* ones in which we should develop fat cells, which means that we should reach our maximum amount after puberty. However, the fat cell has a very accommodating cell wall. It starts out the size of a pen dot and can expand to almost 100 times its size if it needs to store excess fat—great news, right? Thank you, fat cells, for being so accommodating.

And, ladies, it gets worse! Women have different-sized fat cells than men. One study by researchers at Cedars-Sinai Medical Center in L.A. found that women's fat cells are not only larger than men's but are also more efficient at storing fat and holding onto it than the male fat cell. The only difference that researchers could account for was the presence of estrogen in women. Meanwhile, the study found that testosterone stimulates fat cells to break down fat. So men with low testosterone tend to gain weight faster and find it more difficult to lose than their normal-testosterone level counterparts.

After puberty, the average person has between 20 billion and 45 billion fat cells. When you start putting on excess weight, the fat cells begin to expand. Once they have stretched to maximum capacity, and when you do not have any more fat cells left to accommodate the weight, your body makes up the difference: instead of recognizing it is full to capacity—*let's just waste the fat that is now coming in*—it sends signals to neighboring immature mesenchymal stem cells, or "adult" stem cells, to differentiate themselves into more fat cells.

Adult stem cells are in our bodies to develop into muscle, skin tissue, or whatever we need at a given time; if we have an injury, for example, they help us regenerate and heal. But when the fat cells start to signal for the stem cells to differentiate into *more* fat cells, they follow the command. That means the body of an overweight or obese individual can accommodate anywhere from 75 billion and 300 billion fat cells. (As a result, some obese patients have very low muscle mass and poor wound healing capabilities.) And the thing is, once you make fat cells, they hang with you forever. Losing weight shrinks the *size* of the cells, but the total number remains constant. They're your loyal companions. Forever!

Liposuction and surgical resection are the only ways you can rid your body of excess fat cells; you literally have to suck them out or cut them off. Note, however, that liposuction does not in any way improve your overall health. You lose the fat, but the cells left behind still have the ability to signal for more fat cells if you continue your current eating habits and lifestyle. The cells left behind have also retained the ability to receive whatever abnormal signal that caused you to accumulate fat in the first place. So liposuction is not a fix for the problem; it's just one of the ways to get rid of excess cells.

Fat cells not only create signals, but they also produce estrogen and other toxic substances that can interfere with many metabolic processes in the body. One well-studied area is in individuals who have excess visceral fat, which is the fat deposited around the abdominal area. Studies upon studies have shown that these cells secrete metabolically active substances that interfere with liver function, and part of that interference disturbs the liver's ability to regulate blood sugar and cholesterol. This puts you more at risk for diabetes and heart disease. When I counsel patients, I often tell them how important it is to lose the visceral fat because it's a huge health risk on its own, without considering the other harmful conditions obesity can create.

AN UNKNOWN SIGNAL

From all my research and work with overweight or obese patients, the definition for obesity that I have come to accept is: **an abnormal functioning in the weight-control center of the body that causes it to allow accumulation of abnormal amounts of fat, regardless of the degree of food consumption or physical activity.**

This definition acknowledges that the problem is not always the patients' slipups alone. The body itself may also be allowing the accumulation of fat in unhealthy quantities because it has somehow lost its own regulatory mechanisms. The body knows it does not *need* this excess amount of fat, so why does it keep storing it? Many researchers and I believe this happens as a response to a signal that is telling the body to do this. With this modified definition of obesity, the notion of "eat less, exercise more" is not likely to work as a treatment. As long as this unknown signal is present, relentlessly firing commands to your body's weight-control center, you will continue to accumulate excess fat. Eating less and exercising more might slow down the progression, but it cannot ultimately stop the inevitable; net negative daily energy expenditure cannot remove the signal from your body.

Now, do all overweight individuals have this signal?

We all know those people—the ones who can eat whatever they want, whenever they want, and never gain weight. We typically think of them as the "lucky ones," the ones with the "good genes" or "fast metabolism." I believe there is a possibility that these people are "lucky" because they don't have the abnormal signal for excess fat storage the way some of us do.

So, if that is true, then what about those people who *do* lose the weight by eating less and exercising more? I believe that they, like the "lucky" ones, do not have this unknown signal. Their weight problem might very well be the result of overeating and under-exercising. Their bodies consequently would respond to appropriate modifications in diet and lifestyle.

Not everyone is overweight because of overeating. However, I believe it is crucial to understand that not *everyone* is overweight because of overeating. Yes, I agree that a huge percentage of the population is overweight or obese because of bad eating habits, but there are also people who would gain and retain weight regardless. Just like a patient with Cushing's syndrome—a disorder caused by excessive levels of cortisol (a stress hormone) in the blood leading to rapid weight gain—weight gain in individuals with this signal problem has nothing to do with eating or exercise habits. Still, obese patients with Cushing's are often stigmatized as those who are overeating. This stigma causes a delay in diagnosis, prolonging a patient's already frustrating weight loss journey.

Many times, patients come to me weighed down by more than excess fat. "I'm trying to diet," they lament. "I'm exercising. I just can't lose the pounds." I believe individuals who are legitimately doing these things and not finding success probably have a signaling problem that causes their body to accumulate fat, regardless of their efforts to the contrary. I probably experienced this during the three-year period that I struggled to lose my excess pounds. I did *everything* I tell my patients to do, what the medical textbooks ordered, and yet I could not lose the weight or keep it off. I believe a subset of the obese population is struggling from the same condition. We should therefore avoid grouping every overweight individual into the one-size-fits-all category of "obese." Doctors need to remain meticulous about proper diagnosis for all diseases, including this mysterious one called obesity, while the general population needs to guard against judgment.

THE DIAGNOSTIC PROCESS

By now, it should be clear that I don't think it's enough to look at a patient, assess an obvious physical condition, and prescribe cookie-cutter treatments. The patient will only return more disheartened and perhaps with greater weight gain.

There is often a natural course to becoming obese. It starts with 5, 10, or 15 extra pounds. When no action is taken to counter the weight gain, you progress from "pleasantly plump" to mildly overweight to borderline obese. Before you know it, you're morbidly obese and caught in a nasty cycle of health conditions that arise from the disease. When a new patient comes to see me, I have to help trace the path back to the *initial weight gain* before we can place him or her in a defined category. Where did it all begin?

Not surprisingly, I start with food intake. It is a well-known and understood fact that if you eat more calories than you burn, you're going to store the surplus as fat. So, is the patient eating more than he burns? To find out, we go over his diet to find out if he is consuming calorie-dense foods. Economic issues can come into play here, as it's often cheaper to buy not-so-healthy foods. Once diet is determined, what is the patient's typical activity level? Is a sedentary lifestyle the problem?

Let's assume I've found that an average-height overweight patient is consuming a healthy 2,000 calories a day, working out for an hour at least three times a week, and is not losing weight. I would next look to rule out any current or past medical condition, such as endocrine disorders, that might be at play: does the patient have thyroid problems? Is she overproducing cortisol? Or perhaps weight gain is a side effect of a medication she is taking for another condition. For instance, steroids, antidepressants, some seizure medications, and even medicine used to treat diabetes could contribute to weight gain. So, for that matter, could quitting smoking, so I need to ask patients a barrage of lifestyle questions, including about drug and alcohol habits. I also need to know whether a patient is or was recently pregnant, since some hormonal changes that happen during pregnancy can cause women to accumulate more fat afterwards than they did before. And, of course, I must also consider the gender of the patient, since men typically don't accumulate fat as fast as women. On top of all that, I figure a patient's age and metabolism into the equation.

Finally, I factor in genetics. While genetics can contribute to weight gain, this can only be a diagnosis of exclusion: occasionally, strong family history can be a clue, though it is not enough for a diagnosis without evaluating other causes. If I've crossed every other potential cause off the list, I can reasonably suspect that genetics are at play. The fact is that some patients *do* have genetic susceptibility; if both parents are obese, patients have an 80 percent likelihood of becoming obese themselves. So, patients need to know details about their family history when it comes to weight management.

As you can see, an extensive list of factors has to be reviewed with a patient before concluding which group he or she falls into—including the "signal disorder" group. I would estimate that up to 30 percent of my overweight and obese patients fall into this exceptional category. While the percentage of individuals in the true population may not be as high, it's enough for me to say we can't ignore it any longer. There are better answers out there.

CHAPTER 2

HOW DID YOUR **OBESITY BEGIN?**

SOME people gain weight over a short period of time, others over a period of months or years. No matter how long it's taken you to get here, it's probably difficult to trace your way back to the start. How and when did those first few extra pounds turn into 30, 50, 100? You may not know. This makes sense, because chances are, it wasn't just *one thing* that caused your weight gain.

Part of what makes obesity such a complex disease—and treating it effectively so difficult—is that there are so many potential causes. Many experts fall into a particular school of thought regarding obesity, and if they do, they like to insist that their school is *the* school offering the *only* answer. This makes it difficult for obese patients searching for solutions; just when they find one expert in one school of thought claiming answers, another emerges in a different school that wildly contradicts the first. This lack of consistency is overwhelming for someone who's just desperate to know, *How do I lose the weight?*

Most theories fit into one of two major schools of thought—and my goal is to lay them out here in one easily navigable place. Read one theory, read them all, and use the checklists at the end of each description to help pinpoint where your unique case began. Once you start narrowing down what caused your weight gain, we can start building a customized approach to getting you toward your goal!

THEORY 1: YOU ARE EATING TOO MUCH AND NOT EXERCISING ENOUGH

Okay, so maybe the mantra of "eat less, exercise more" actually applies to you; it does for more than half of obese patients. These individuals are eating more than their daily recommended calories and are not exercising enough to make up for the difference.

Now, here's where misconceptions can happen. The number of calories you need each day to maintain your weight is actually highly specific. It depends on your gender, current weight, height, age, muscle mass and level of physical activity. A quick Internet search for "Harris-Benedict equation" will give you the information you need to calculate first your basal metabolic rate (BMR)—or the amount of energy you expend while at rest to sustain your basic life functions—and then your total daily calorie requirements. But if you'd like to calculate this now, here's what to do:

1. Find your BMR.

Men: BMR = 66 + (6.23 x weight in pounds) + (12.7 x height in inches) - (6.76 x age in years)

Women: BMR = 655 + (4.35 x weight in pounds) + (4.7 x height in inches) - (4.7 x age in years)

So, for example, this is my BMR calculation:

655 + (783) + (338.4) - (150.4) = 1,626

Now for the rest of the equation.

2. Incorporate how much you exercise.

Little to no exercise:
Daily calories needed = BMR x 1.2

Light exercise (1–3 days per week):
Daily calories needed = BMR x 1.375

Moderate exercise (3–5 days per week):
Daily calories needed = BMR x 1.55

Heavy exercise (6–7 days per week):
Daily calories needed = BMR x 1.725

Very heavy exercise (2 times per day):
Daily calories needed = BMR x 1.9

So, my total daily calories needed = 1,626 x 1.375, or **2,235.** This is the amount of calories I need to maintain my weight at my current activity level.

It's very important to know the amount of calories you need each day. First, determining this number should go a long way in helping you figure out whether you are, indeed, "eating too much." If you know your body needs 2,500 calories to maintain its current weight and you *also* know you're consuming twice that, you can live in denial no longer. On the other hand, if you're consuming *less* than your daily required calories and either not losing weight or still gaining weight, it's likely that something else is at work. Note, however, that the Harris-Benedict equation is not perfect. It's a "guestimate," especially because it does not take muscle mass into consideration. But it's a start. It is better, in my opinion, than the magical 2,000 calories we're all told we need to eat daily.

Now, let's not neglect the second part of this theory—exercise.

Why is exercise so important? Exercise increases the energy demand on the body. As you've already seen, the amount of exercise you get on a regular basis plays into your BMR, which determines how many daily calories you need to maintain your weight. Exercise *also* determines your metabolic age, which is found by comparing your BMR against that of others in your own chronological age group. (Again, do a quick search online for "metabolic age calculator" to learn where you stand.) Ideally, your metabolic age should be less than or equal to your actual chronological age, but I find that for a lot of overweight and obese patients, metabolic age is usually way higher than it should be. An overweight woman, for example, might have a metabolic age of 52 even though her chronological age is only 37. That tells me her body thinks it's much older than it is, and therefore her cells slow down their metabolism to match that of a 52-year-old. This is why only exercise decreases the metabolic age; weight loss in itself does not.

Now, what counts as "exercise?" Some patients think working a physically demanding job means they exercise. "I go up and down the stairs all day every day," one patient tells me. Another says, "I stock shelves at a Wal-Mart—I'm busy climbing ladders and lifting boxes for hours!" Overweight patients whose work requires this kind of activity rarely exercise when they get home. "I'm dead tired," they say. "I feel like I exercise all day!" Others tell me they "exercise" by chasing their young kids around. "Isn't that enough?" they ask.

I understand the frustration and exhaustion, but the short answer is no, it's not enough.

Exercise is, by definition, an activity that increases your heart rate and keeps it there for at least 20 minutes. For example, moderate exercise should cause you to break a sweat after about 10 minutes of engaging in it non-stop. Your breathing should become deeper, more frequent. You can carry on a conversation but would not be able to sing if you tried. The CDC recommends 150 minutes of *this* type of exercise each week; if you're not putting in this amount of time, under this definition of exercise, then you're not doing enough physical activity. Period.

CHECKLIST

☑ Do you consume more than your total daily required calories, as determined by the Harris-Benedict equation?

☑ Do you eat more than you need to fulfill your hunger?

☑ Do you have difficulty determining when you are actually full?

☑ Do you eat on the go or in front of the TV (also known as mindless eating)?

☑ Do you have the habit of cleaning off your plate even when you are full?

☑ Do you put off exercise more than you actually engage in it?

☑ Are you too busy or exhausted to exercise?

☑ Do you drink extra caffeinated drinks for energy to pull you through the day?

If you answered yes to most of these questions, it's possible that this theory explains your weight gain. It did for me. I gained the weight when I stopped exercising and watching what I was eating. But it wasn't the whole story, as it may not be for you. After all, if obesity were as simple as this theory, we should all be able to lose weight the minute we reverse the action—once we start eating less and exercising more—but that's often not the case. So what else could be going on?

YOUR FOOD CONTENT IS CAUSING YOUR WEIGHT GAIN

It may be that you're eating only three times a day, but what you're ingesting is highly dense in calories—in which case, you may not be eating *too much* but eating all the wrong foods. You know those foods, those highly palatable and irresistible ones: the cheeseburgers, the French fries, the fried chicken. The fast food, the desserts. The cheap food. Reaching for it is a habit for a large portion of the population.

Most of these high-calorie foods are foods with very high glycemic index (GI) or glycemic load (GL). The GI measures how fast a particular food and portion size, respectively, affect your blood sugar and insulin levels. Glucose, which is used as the reference standard, has a GI index of 100. Any food with a GI greater than 70 is high, while an index less than 55 is considered low. High GI foods break down too quickly during digestion, converting easily to simple sugars such as glucose and releasing them rapidly into the bloodstream. One good example is white bread, which is wheat that has been bleached and processed and now is just a simple sugar, with no nutritional value. As soon as it hits the bloodstream, it makes your blood sugar spike, triggering a second hunger response soon after. Low GI foods break down more slowly, releasing glucose gradually. Glycemic load, meanwhile, determines the quality of the carbohydrate in a particular portion of food. A GL number greater than 20 is high, while less than 10 is considered low. There is compelling evidence that high GI/GL foods are associated with increased risk of obesity, diabetes, and heart disease.

GLYCEMIC INDEX AND GLYCEMIC LOAD OF SOME COMMON FOODS

FOOD	Glycemic index (glucose=100)	Serving size (grams)	Glycemic load per serving
BAKERY PRODUCTS AND BREADS			
Banana cake, made with sugar	47±8	80	18
Banana cake, made without sugar	55±10	80	16
Sponge cake, plain	46±6	63	17
Vanilla cake made from packet mix with vanilla frosting (Betty Crocker)	42±4	111	24
Waffles, Aunt Jemima (Quaker Oats)	76	35	10
Bagel, white, frozen	72	70	25
Baguette, white, plain	95±15	30	15
Coarse barley bread, 75–80% kernels, average	34±4	30	7
Hamburger bun	61	30	9
Kaiser roll	73	30	12
Pumpernickel bread	50±4	30	6
50% cracked wheat kernel bread	58	30	12
White wheat flour bread	70±0	30	10
Wonder™ bread, average	73±2	30	10
Whole wheat bread, average	71± 2	30	9
100% Whole Grain™ bread (Natural Ovens)	51±11	30	7
Pita bread, white	57	30	10

FOOD	Glycemic index (glucose=100)	Serving size (grams)	Glycemic load per serving
Corn tortilla	52	50	12
Wheat tortilla	30	50	8

BEVERAGES/DRINKS			
Coca Cola®, average	58±5	250	15
Fanta®, orange soft drink	68±6	250	23
Lucozade®, original (sparkling glucose drink)	95±10	250	40
Apple juice, unsweetened, average	40±1	250	12
Cranberry juice cocktail (Ocean Spray®)	68±3	250	24
Grapefruit juice, unsweetened	48	250	11
Orange juice, average	50±4	250	13
Tomato juice, canned	38±4	250	4

BREAKFAST CEREALS AND RELATED PRODUCTS			
All-Bran™, average	42±5	30	4
Coco Pops™, average	77	30	20
Cornflakes™, average	81±3	30	21
Cream of Wheat™ (Nabisco)	66	250	17
Cream of Wheat™, Instant (Nabisco)	74	250	22
Grapenuts™, average	71±4	30	15
Muesli, average	66±9	30	16
Oatmeal, average	58±4	250	13
Instant oatmeal, average	66±1	250	17
Puffed wheat, average	74±7	30	16
Raisin Bran™ (Kellogg's)	61±5	30	12
Special K™ (Kellogg's)	69±5	30	14

GRAINS			
Pearled barley, average	25±1	150	11
Sweet corn on the cob, average	53±4	150	17

FOOD	Glycemic index (glucose=100)	Serving size (grams)	Glycemic load per serving
Couscous, average	65±4	150	23
White rice, average	64±7	150	23
Quick cooking white basmati	60±5	150	23
Brown rice, average	55±5	150	18
Converted, white rice (Uncle Ben's®)	38	150	14
Whole wheat kernels, average	41±3	50	14
Bulgur, average	48±2	150	12

COOKIES AND CRACKERS			
Graham crackers	74	25	14
Vanilla wafers	77	25	14
Shortbread	64±8	25	10
Rice cakes, average	78±9	25	17
Rye crisps, average	64±2	25	11
Soda crackers	74	25	12

DAIRY PRODUCTS AND ALTERNATIVES			
Ice cream, regular	61±7	50	8
Ice cream, premium	37±3	50	4
Milk, full fat	27±4	250	3
Milk, skim	32±5	250	4
Reduced-fat yogurt with fruit, average	27±1	200	7

FRUITS			
Apple, average	38±2	120	6
Banana, ripe	51	120	13
Dates, dried	103±21	60	42
Grapefruit	25	120	3
Grapes, average	46±3	120	8
Orange, average	42±3	120	5
Peach, average	42±14	120	5

FOOD	Glycemic index (glucose=100)	Serving size (grams)	Glycemic load per serving
Peach, canned in light syrup	52	120	9
Pear, average	38±2	120	4
Pear, canned in pear juice	44	120	5
Prunes, pitted	29±4	60	10
Raisins	64±11	60	28
Watermelon	72±13	120	4

BEANS AND NUTS			
Baked beans, average	48±8	150	7
Black eyed peas, average	42±9	150	13
Black beans	30	150	7
Chickpeas, average	28±6	150	8
Chickpeas, canned in brine	42	150	9
Navy beans, average	38±6	150	12
Kidney beans, average	28±4	150	7
Lentils, average	29±1	150	5
Soy beans, average	18±3	150	1
Cashews, salted	22±5	50	3
Peanuts, average	14±8	50	1

PASTA AND NOODLES			
Fettucini, average	40±8	180	18
Macaroni, average	47±2	180	23
Macaroni and Cheese (Kraft)	64	180	32
Spaghetti, white, boiled 5 min, average	38±3	180	18
Spaghetti, white, boiled 20 min, average	61±3	180	27
Spaghetti, wholemeal, boiled, average	37±5	180	16

FOOD	Glycemic index (glucose=100)	Serving size (grams)	Glycemic load per serving
SNACKS			
Corn chips, plain, salted, average	63±10	50	17
Fruit Roll-Ups®	99±12	30	24
M & M's®, peanut	33±3	30	6
Microwave popcorn, plain, average	72±17	20	8
Potato chips, average	54±3	50	11
Pretzels, oven-baked	83±9	30	16
Snickers Bar®	55±14	60	19

FOOD	Glycemic index (glucose=100)	Serving size (grams)	Glycemic load per serving
VEGETABLES			
Green peas, average	48±5	80	3
Carrots, average	47±16	80	3
Parsnips	97±19	80	12
Baked russet potato, average	85±12	150	26
Boiled white potato, average	50±9	150	14
Instant mashed potato, average	85±3	150	17
Sweet potato, average	61±7	150	17
Yam, average	37±8	150	13

FOOD	Glycemic index (glucose=100)	Serving size (grams)	Glycemic load per serving
MISCELLANEOUS			
Hummus (chickpea salad dip)	6±4	30	0
Chicken nuggets, frozen, reheated in microwave oven 5 min	46±4	100	7
Pizza, plain baked dough, served with parmesan cheese and tomato sauce	80	100	22
Pizza, Super Supreme (Pizza Hut)	36±6	100	9
Honey, average	55±5	25	10

The complete list of the glycemic index and glycemic load for 750 foods can be found in the article "International tables of glycemic index and glycemic load values: 2002," by Kaye Foster-Powell, Susanna H.A. Holt, and Janette C. Brand-Miller in the July 2002 American Journal of Clinical Nutrition, Vol. 62, pages 5–56.

THE CARBS CONUNDRUM

In the last few years, the reputation of carbs has been complicated past sense. You read one headline stating that carbs are making us fat; then you turn around and hear carbs can lower risk of chronic disease. So which is it, good or bad? Actually, it's both.

Good carbs—or carbohydrates high in fiber—are essential nutrients, just like lean proteins, fatty acids, vitamins, minerals, and water. With low GI/GL numbers, they have a role in every healthy diet. Some cells in our bodies, such as red blood cells and brain cells, specifically require the glucose obtained from good carbs for energy. Examples of good carbs are whole grains, vegetables, fruits, and beans. Bad carbs, on the other hand, are those refined and processed carbohydrates that strip away beneficial fiber and nutrients. Examples: white bread, white rice, and candy. See more examples in the GI/GL list.

So, are you eating foods that are counteracting your efforts to lose weight?

CHECKLIST

☑ Are you mostly eating on the run or in your car?

☑ Do you eat out at restaurants because you hate cooking?

☑ Are you eating mostly highly palatable or highly irresistible foods?

☑ Are you the type that can't say no when you are offered free food or super-sized meals?
(Heck, you think, *for just 50 cents more ...!)*

If you answered yes to most of these questions, it's possible that the *content* of your food, in addition to or instead of the amount, has contributed to your weight gain.

YOU ARE AN EMOTIONAL EATER

Okay, so maybe you're eating too much or eating all the wrong foods. Why?

Emotional eating can play a role in weight gain. In my experience, it played a *major* role. I gained weight during a period of time when I was stressed and depressed but refused to seek help. I was more worried about the stigma of being treated for a psychiatric disorder than the effect it was having on my overall health. To be honest, if I had seen someone about it, I might have saved myself dozens of pounds and a lot of heartache.

I graduated from the University of Maryland in 2000 with a degree in biochemistry and decided to work for a couple of years before going to medical school. I ended up doing drug development and research for a pharmaceutical company. I packed a lunch for work so I didn't have to eat from the cafeteria or give in to fast food temptations. I steered clear of the vending machines and avoided the extras around the break room (the candy, the leftover cheesecake from someone's birthday). Taking it a step further, I purposely didn't bring money to work so that I would not be able to go out to eat with my colleagues. Even then, though, I had a weakness: Breyers Vanilla Bean Ice Cream. I don't know what it is about that stuff, but I can't just enjoy a serving or two; I have to eat the whole box. In fact, I will not buy it anymore. I know that once I buy it, I'm going to eat it all. No self-control.

Despite my Breyers habit, however, I was able to maintain my weight. Once I was in medical school in Virginia, I rode my bike to school—which was a mile away—another mile to the gym to work out for an hour, and then back home. That was my daily routine. Because I didn't like to cook, it would have been easy to just pop something in the microwave each night, but I never liked frozen dinners or the taste of processed foods—and rarely went to the grocery store—so my diet mostly consisted of oatmeal. I ate oatmeal for breakfast, sometimes oatmeal for lunch, and sometimes oatmeal for dinner. If I got sick of it, I added some flavor with cranberries or raisins. When my mom came to visit, she prepared and froze home-cooked African foods for me, so that was where the variety in my diet came from. Other than that, I was on the oatmeal diet for most of medical school, which—in addition to my exercise—made it very easy for me to maintain my weight of 160.

After medical school, I started a relationship that quickly became very serious—we got engaged. But then I ended up breaking off the engagement, and I spiraled into major depression. At that point, everything I knew about diet and exercise went out the window. I was so depressed and emotional that I just didn't care what I looked like. I know exactly what Britney Spears went though when she decided to shave off all her hair; I cut off my own hair to try to express some of what I was feeling. My family was shocked, but I felt as if I had control over some part of my life.

The relief didn't last long.

I started eating more to fill the void my breakup had left behind. I ate a lot more. I ate alone. I ate late. I ate anything.

I was definitely off the oatmeal diet. Exercise went out the window. I ate more carbs, more fat, more sugar, and more salt. The more I ate, the more I craved. I ate chips and then more chips. Then I ate eat ice cream and maybe some bread. I was not even thinking about what I was putting into my body. My depression was more powerful than my ability to reason about what I was physically doing to myself. I didn't like what I saw in the mirror, but I didn't care.

My mother was concerned and tried to help me face my depression and get help, but I didn't want to talk to her or anyone else. By the time I realized what was happening, my weight had reached around 190. I had gained 30 pounds within a year. That was when my father began teasing me. He is usually a very reserved man and would never comment on a woman's weight, but he started calling me "Big Momma." That was a reality check for me.

It was around this time that my husband came into my life. I had met him while I was in college and had known him for more than eight years, and he never mentioned anything to me about my weight. He was simply interested in starting a relationship with me, though I was not ready to begin one at that time. Even though my father's comments made me realize what I was doing to myself, I continued to eat and gain. By the time my husband and I were married in 2008, I was around 205 pounds.

I got pregnant right away, and that, combined with being in residency, was exhausting. I worked 30 hours straight with no break, went home and grabbed eight hours of sleep, and then headed back to work. It was a high stress situation—newly married, pregnant, residency, messed-up sleeping cycle—and my body was reacting to all of this.

My coping mechanism? You guessed it. I ate. My weight ballooned to 240 pounds.

I should have seen someone who could have helped me cope with my emotions, but at least my experience gives me insight into my patients' emotional struggles around their weight gain. I see, often before they do, how they stuff themselves with food to avoid confronting anger, resentment, fear, frustration, boredom, or loneliness—and it works for a while. That's because we usually reach for the salty, sugary, fatty foods, which release chemicals called neurotransmitters into the bloodstream. They trigger the reward center in our brain just like cocaine does for an addict. However, once the neurotransmitters are reabsorbed, we're left feeling down again. The food euphoria has disappeared, just like the cocaine high. So we eat more of these foods to capture the feeling again and again. In the meantime, the original emotions are now amplified by the physical effects of the overeating. It's a nasty cycle that's difficult to break.

So, how do you know that you might be an emotional eater?

CHECKLIST

☑ Do you overeat when you are stressed?

☑ Is your overeating triggered by some major life event?

☑ Do you turn to salty foods and sweet foods mainly when you're stressed?

☑ Do you eat even when you're not hungry?

☑ Do you continue eating even when you feel comfortably full?

☑ Do you snack more when you're alone?

☑ Do you eat more when you're at home compared to when you're at work or outdoors?

☑ Are you snacking at certain times of the day, mostly at night?

☑ Do you feel hungry in your *stomach* or in your *head?*

☑ Do you feel guilty after eating?

A majority of resounding "yes" answers indicate that you're probably an emotional eater.

THEORY 2: YOUR GENETICS HAVE CAUSED YOU TO GAIN WEIGHT

Some patients say that the reason they're obese is because it runs in their family. Actually, a lot of studies out there support this: if both your parents are obese, you have up to an 80 percent chance of being obese, while if both your parents are thin, there is only a 10 percent chance that you will be obese. More than 30 published studies have looked at this issue and estimate that the heritability of one's BMI ranges between 60–80 percent after adjusting for other factors. So, yes, genetics can *predispose* you to obesity, but does it *doom* you to it?

Theoretically, identical twins get all their genetics from the same pool. Studies of adopted twins who were raised by different sets of parents have found that 40–80 percent of the time, if one twin is obese, the other is, too. The different environments don't seem to matter, supporting the strength of the genetics argument. Then again, 40–80 percent of the time is not 100 percent of the time, which says that other factors can play a role. So, even if you have two obese parents, you are not guaranteed to be obese—you have at *least* a 20 percent chance of not becoming obese.

Many genetic syndromes can influence weight. One in particular worth mentioning is called Prader-Willi syndrome (PWS). Occurring in every 15,000 births, and equally between males and females, it is the most common genetic reason for childhood obesity. It happens when part or all of a particular chromosome—specifically chromosome 15—on the father's side is missing. This causes the child to become obese no matter how strict a diet he follows or how much exercise he does. While there is no cure for PWS, there are ways to treat some of the symptoms, such as the insatiable appetite.

Another possible hereditary reason for obesity is known as the "thrifty metabolism gene." A geneticist named James V. Neel suggested that we have certain genes that *used to be* helpful to us in certain conditions but are now detrimental. For example, the only way people survived long periods of famine was by their genes adapting to that environment, slowing their metabolism to allow them to go without food. Though culture and technology can change quickly, evolution is slow. Some of our genes, Mr. Neel proposes, haven't evolved as fast, and now they are functioning in an environment of excess and easy assess to high-calorie foods. No wonder there's an imbalance!

An example of this theory in action can be seen in the Pima Indians, who live mostly in New Mexico and Arizona. This group has been studied quite often because it survived the harsh Sonoran Desert (one of the largest and hottest deserts in North America). Researchers think it is because they carry the thrifty gene, which allowed them to metabolize food more efficiently when supply was low. Now, in an environment where there is access to food all the time, this population has the highest percentage of obesity prevalence. It's possible, therefore, that the same genes that used to work for them are now working against them.

THE METABOLISM QUESTION

You may have heard that the reason you keep gaining weight or can't lose weight is because you have a slow metabolism. Sound familiar?

There is so much conflicting information about this theory. You see it all the time, maybe online or in magazines— "Obesity Caused by Slow Metabolism." The next day's headline is "Obesity NOT Explained by Slow Metabolism." One day, you might read that thin people have high metabolism, and the next, you read how their metabolism is the same as an obese person's. Everyone does their own research and concludes something different, and all refer to it as *metabolism*. So how much of a role does metabolism actually play?

Metabolism is a process by which the body breaks down food and converts it into energy, either for use or for storage. Metabolism is a process by which the body breaks down food and converts it into energy, either for use or for storage. It's the total sum of all the work of our chemical factories (the cells). They take calories from food and transform it into energy called ATP. Cells need ATP to carry out their daily functions. The total amount of food calories needed for the cells to sustain life is what we call basal metabolic rate. This is the same BMR calculation we estimated earlier in this chapter.

A high metabolic rate means that your body requires a lot of energy to get its job done. When your metabolic rate is low, that means it does *not* need a lot of energy to sustain itself. Therefore, the argument in the metabolism school is that someone with a low BMR requirement will gain weight through excess fat storage if they eat the same amount of calories as someone with a higher BMR requirement.

A lot plays into the metabolism equation. Your genes have a lot to do with your metabolism, as do your weight, age, gender, activity level, muscle mass, and how frequently you eat. Also, your underlying health and nutritional choices play a role. For example, males generally have more muscle and testosterone than women, while women generally carry less muscle, less testosterone, and a little more fat than men. This goes to show why, pound for pound, women tend to have a slightly slower metabolism than men.

As far as the validity of metabolic rate in obesity goes, there is confusing information from researchers. For example, a 2003 article in *Lancet,* a well-known medical journal, presented a study arguing that dieting slows down your metabolism. This suggests, therefore, that it's easier to gain weight after you diet—wonderful news for those of us who have tried dieting for years, right? But yet an article in *JAMA* said no, dieting doesn't lower your BMR—your BMR is lower after you lose weight because that is the new rate your lower body weight requires! So, which one is right? Well, my question about the *Lancet* article is: did dieting *really* lower the BMR, or was the BMR too high to start with due to the excess weight? If you look at the Harris-Benedict equation closely, you will see that current body weight is one of the numbers plugged into the equation to arrive at BMR. Therefore, the lower BMR after dieting doesn't mean that your body is now less efficient; it just uses less energy at the new low weight, making more sense of the latter study in *JAMA.*

Some of the women I see say that their weight problem hit when they reached a certain age—say, 35—and they believe their metabolism must have slowed at that point. There is some truth to the age correlation, but it has to do with the fact that we lose some muscle as we age unless we actively work to keep the muscle mass up. Muscle burns calories, even when it's just sitting there not doing anything—so when you start to lose that, sure, your metabolism will go, too.

So, can genetics play a role in obesity, whether through predisposition, inherited disorders, and/or metabolism? Why, yes. But it is far too complex for us to come to a simple conclusion about how it causes us to gain (or not gain) weight. As a physician, I can only say someone is obese secondary to genetics after eliminating all other possible causes (again, a diagnosis of exclusion). So, if you've nixed the other theories I've discussed, you should ask yourself the following:

CHECKLIST

☑ Are any or a majority of your first-degree relatives (mother, father, siblings) also obese?

☑ Are you a twin; if so, are you an identical twin?

☑ If you are an identical twin, is your identical twin also obese?

☑ Have you been overweight as far back as you can remember?

☑ Have you *truly* tried dieting and exercising, as laid out in this book, without any success?

If you answered mostly "yes" to these questions—and mostly no to the others in this chapter—it's possible that genetics are causing your obesity. However, can you blame them entirely? I don't think so.

CHAPTER 3

ENVIRONMENT AND CULTURE: COULD THEY BE THE CULPRITS?

BEFORE 1980, the rate of obesity in the U.S. was feeble: around 12 percent. By 1980, however, a researcher at the CDC noticed a sudden jump in the obesity rate. Many speculate that these causes must be environmental, because— as we know—genes couldn't have changed so quickly.

One of the only things researchers could pinpoint as changing, at least in the U.S., was the environment. Fast food restaurants proliferated, portion sizes increased, drinks were highly sweetened, and foods became calorie-dense with low nutritional value. The culture also changed—more families were (and are) dining out, as opposed to the days when mothers stayed home and cooked. It was more common then for kids to eat breakfast at home and pack their lunch for school, and now it is not that way all the time.

So what is the obsession with food in our society? Is there a reason that a large amount of the population tends to overeat? Researchers have found that we are probably "addicted" to food, and many people blame it on the food industry. The food industry has mastered the art of making food that triggers our brain's reward center. They believe that foods high in fat, sugar, and salt in a certain combination can stimulate the same part of the brain that is affected by illegal drugs. As with drugs, our brains continue to think of those foods even after we're done eating. That sense of yearning is what keeps us going back for more.

In a book called *The End of Overeating,* Dr. David Kessler interviewed food industry insiders who blatantly admitted to making money by creating addictive foods. Studies have shown that when made "right," these foods increase the dopamine levels in the brain in a way comparable to doing cocaine! Amazing! So for some, food *can* be a drug of choice.

Is everyone equally susceptible to food addiction? Dr. Kessler concluded that some of us are more genetically predisposed than others. You might compare this to the way one person can experiment with drugs and walk away while another becomes immediately hooked. The food industry has made it a science to target the latter demographic, but it has an effect on everyone.

I moved to the U.S. to be with my parents after finishing high school. At 16 years old, I was around 5 feet 10 inches tall and weighed about 125 pounds, with a BMI around 18. I wasn't vigilant about checking my weight, but people viewed me as thin. In Nigerian culture at the time, men actually preferred women who had a little bit of meat on them, so to them, I was skinny.

Once in the U.S., I started college at the University of Maryland. I also worked part-time at a fast food restaurant called Philly's Steak Express. I was a cashier but sometimes helped with food prep, so my exposure to American food began while working there. I wasn't crazy about the food, so I ate fairly little of it, but I put on a few pounds anyway.

At home, where I lived with my parents and siblings, we mostly ate a Nigerian diet—usually a home-cooked meal containing healthy portions of carbs, proteins (such as beef or chicken), and a lot of sauces. Unlike American sauces, which tend to be heavy and high in fat content, Nigerian sauces are mostly tomato-based and more like soups. These sauces and foods were served over rice and often with bread or yams, which have higher fiber content than potatoes. I continued to eat most meals at home, even while working in the fast food restaurant, because that is what the Nigerian community does.

After living in the U.S. for a while, I noticed that people were not calling me "thin" anymore. I assumed it was because I'd started eating more of the American diet when I wasn't at home, and I was driving more than walking, but my weight gain didn't bother me. My clothes actually fit better, and I was happy. By this time, I weighed around 160 pounds—about 35 pounds heavier than when I'd arrived in the U.S. four years earlier.

Around then, I took a college course on nutrition and exercise, and it was the first time I realized I needed to exercise and watch what I ate. That was where I first learned about fat cells. I began paying more attention to my weight, exercising and watching what I was eating. I remember looking at my relatives—my parents, aunts, and uncles—who had been in the United States for a while, and noticing how much weight they had put on. Of course, I never would have mentioned it to them, but I hoped I could keep myself from gaining as much as they had.

Meanwhile, my family noticed the subtle change in me around food. At gatherings where they ate foods I thought were fattening, I reached for salads or fruits. "Why are you eating rabbit food?" they teased. To them, I was still thin and probably too conscious of my weight, but I didn't mind. At six feet tall and with a BMI still around 21–22, I was comfortable with my body but aware that my new American environment could sneak up on me if I wasn't careful.

Another argument for environmental causes is the fact that we see a huge difference in weight based on whether you are living in a low-income or high-income environment. High-income neighborhoods often have access to parks and trails and health foods stores, whereas in low-income neighborhoods, physical activity is often limited because parks are far away or inaccessible. In these cases, the television becomes the main form of entertainment, and there tend to be poorer food choices based on what individuals can afford. Children growing up in this type of environment will most often pick up the habits and culture of those around them, contributing to the childhood obesity rates.

In medical school, one of my colleagues noted that when she was living in a high-income neighborhood, she was always conscious of her weight because everyone around her was thinner than she was. She kept an eye on her calorie intake, went to the gym, and attempted to lead an overall healthy lifestyle. When she could no longer afford the rent there, she moved to a less expensive area of town

... and then she noticed that she was gaining weight. The grocery stores around her new apartment didn't stock the organic and healthy foods, and she was no longer as conscious of her weight because she was actually thinner than those around her in the new neighborhood.

To me, these are pretty convincing arguments. So, could your environment be playing a role in your weight gain?

CHECKLIST

☑ Did your weight gain start when you moved from a higher-income neighborhood to a lower-income neighborhood?

☑ Did your weight gain start when your income level decreased?

☑ Did you change your food choices from healthy to what you could more easily afford?

☑ Did your weight gain start when you moved from another country to the U.S.?

☑ Did your weight gain start when job conditions changed and it became easier to eat out than stay in? Drive rather than walk everywhere?

YOUR CULTURE AND YOUR WEIGHT

Back in the eighteenth and nineteenth centuries, being overweight or obese was viewed positively in many cultures. It was considered a sign of health, wealth, beauty, and prosperity. In the late 1800s to early 1900s, a group known as the New England Fat Men's Club was made up of men who were obviously overweight and had large girth (potbellies). The cultural view of them was that they must be rich—and a lot of them *were* rich!—because eating enough to create the required excess poundage cost a fair amount of money. As a result, women looked at these men more favorably—if a man was in that club, he must be wealthy and ideal for marrying.

Though this cultural view seems antiquated or bizarre to most Americans today, it still exists in different parts of the world. In Africa, as I mentioned, men prefer women who are curvier. Some Arab populations, such as Mauritania, encourage "wife fattening," and parents send their young girls to "fat camps," where they are force-fed so they look more plump and prosperous to potential husbands.

While less extreme, this phenomenon also occurs in cultures within the U.S. I've seen this often in Hispanic communities, where parents and grandparents show off their overweight children as if to say, "I feed them well." There is a certain amount of pride—especially in lower-income families—that comes with being able to keep children "well-fed" enough for them to be overweight.

Meanwhile, the types of foods in certain cultures are obesogenic—a recently coined medical term referring to factors that cause weight gain. In some areas, the way that foods are cooked and what is considered tasty varies. In the South, for instance, "tasty" foods are cooked in high fat, heavy creams, and sugar. Southern foods are often layered; you get your batter, dip the chicken, deep fry it, then you pour gumbo or some type of sweet sauce on it. Southerners consider these types of foods part of their culture.

Some cultures also encourage eating through frequent social gatherings. Hispanic and African-American communities, for example, are very family-oriented and promote togetherness through social events. Often in these settings, they prepare excess amounts of food, and it's sometimes considered insulting not to at least *try* everything. (And trust me, there's no such thing as just "trying" everything.) The result is weight gain over time, possibly before you even realize it.

If your culture is contributing to your weight gain, it may actually be having a negative impact on your overall health. If you suspect that your culture might be a culprit, ask yourself the following questions:

CHECKLIST

☑ Does your culture promote activities that mostly involve food/eating?

☑ Does your culture promote the type of cooking that is high in fat or "layered"?

☑ Does your culture ignore exercise as a way of life?

☑ Do you find it hard to stick to your diet or lifestyle change because you would offend one or more family members?

☑ Do your relatives consider it rude for you not to eat whatever "delicacy" they bring to events?

If you answered mostly yes to these questions, it's likely that your culture is a contributing factor to your weight gain.

CHAPTER 4

HEALTH EFFECTS
OF OBESITY

OKAY—I hope that by now you've begun to narrow down possible culprits to your weight gain. But a part of you may still be wondering, *What is* really *wrong with having a few extra pounds?* Western society stigmatizes "fat," yes, but why? Why shouldn't we embrace our extra padding and be comfortable with who we are?

I'll be the first to champion being confident in your skin and finding your *own* ideal weight and body shape. (Size 0 just isn't realistic—or healthy—for most of us.) But the reality is that excess weight can lead to life-altering and even life-threatening health conditions. *Time* magazine recently reported that being just 40 pounds overweight can increase your risk of:

- Heart attack by 360 percent
- Cancer by 80 percent
- High blood pressure (hypertension) by 266 percent
- Type II diabetes by 2,060 percent
- Arthritis by 400 percent
- Dying sooner by 110 percent

The last statistic is usually my first warning for patients.

SHORTENED LIFE SPAN

Obese patients live an average of 10 years less than normal-weight people their age. This has been well documented in sumo wrestlers, an interesting group of people whose job it is to gain weight as fast as they can and maintain it over a long period of time. (Very different from most people's goals!) Even though sumo wrestlers exercise, they overeat, consuming around 20,000 calories a day. They wake up, go to the gym, and work out for five hours on an empty stomach. By the time they finish, it's lunchtime and they're starving. Lunch consists of at least 10,000 calories of food, and immediately after eating, they settle in for a nap. After sleeping for between two and four hours, they hit up another 10,000 calories for dinner. Can you imagine what a 10,000-calorie meal looks like? That's like eating 10 double cheeseburgers, large fries, and the largest soda at a fast food chain. After their dinner of high-calorie, fatty processed carbs, the sumo wrestlers return to bed for the night having gained an average of 5 to 10 pounds, and they repeat the same routine the next day. Once they gain all the weight they want or need, they must try to maintain it; that is the sport. But it is also a health risk: sumo wrestlers live, on average, 10 years less than the average Japanese male.

What actually contributes to this shortened lifespan? What *is* it about obesity that causes such strain on the body's internal organs and systems? And is it possible that you're already suffering from an obesity-related disorder without realizing or admitting it?

A female patient of mine came in to the exam room and said, "Doc, I know I have weight problems, but I'm only here today because of my knee. It won't stop bothering me." After taking her medical history and examining her, I found that she had crepitus in both knees, which is when your cartilage has rubbed away in the joint space and bone is starting to grate against bone. In her case, it was the beginning of early onset arthritis. My patient cried at the diagnosis, telling me that her grandmother had really bad arthritis and it limited everything she did. My patient had mentioned her pain to her grandmother before coming to see me, and her grandmother said, "That sounds like Arthur," which was what she called arthritis. My patient thought she was too young to have that, so she brushed her grandmother off. When she asked me, "Why am I getting arthritis?" I had to be honest: it was most likely the excess 200 pounds she was carrying. Could her arthritis be genetic? Maybe, but as long as she was still overweight, there was no way to tell for sure. My patient cried even more when she recalled that her grandma had said, "Arthur does not discriminate against age, sex, or color."

I see this a lot—patients coming to me seeking help for the effect, not the cause. In a society that values quick fixes and cure-alls, it's not surprising for people to hope for a diagnosis—and a pill—that will help their joints feel better, help them sleep better at night, help them get pregnant and have healthy babies. It's less overwhelming than coping with the need to lose 20 or 50 or 200 pounds, but this is *not* a case where denial will serve you well. I want to educate you not only on what diseases are associated with obesity, but also *why*. I hope once the relationship between cause and effect is made clearer, you'll embark (or continue) on your weight loss journey with even greater purpose.

HIGH BLOOD PRESSURE

What we consider high blood pressure or hypertension is when the heart is pumping blood against arterial pressure that is higher than what is considered "normal." An example of normal arterial pressure is 120/80 in an adult: the systolic number on the top is derived from how much pressure is generated when the heart contracts while the diastolic number on the bottom comes from when the heart relaxes. One or both of these numbers can be high. Hypertension is diagnosed when the blood pressure reads 140/90 or more on at least two separate occasions.

An overweight person has more body tissue (particularly more fat tissue) to supply with blood. To accomplish this, the blood volume must increase. With more blood in the arteries, a higher pressure is generated, and the heart has to pump harder and harder against this pressure to meet demand. When a patient loses excess weight, blood pressure often lowers right along with the numbers on the scale.

Hypertension is often called "The Silent Killer" because even though one in three adult Americans has it, they have no symptoms. Longstanding untreated high blood pressure can cause major havoc. It can damage arteries (causing arteriosclerosis—sometimes called hardening of the arteries—or aneurysms); damage kidneys (causing renal failure and need for dialysis); damage the heart (causing heart attack, enlarged heart, or heart failure); and/or damage the brain (causing strokes or vascular dementia). Decreasing weight, salt intake, alcohol intake, and stress; increasing exercise; and quitting smoking improves blood pressure numbers.

HIGH CHOLESTEROL

Cholesterol, a waxy substance produced by the liver and also found in certain foods, is needed to make cell walls, some hormones (e.g., testosterone), and certain vitamins (vitamin D), and to create bile salts (which help digest fat). The liver produces about 75 percent of the total body cholesterol, which is about 1,000 milligrams of cholesterol per day. We probably consume another 150 to 250 milligrams in the foods we eat daily. Besides making cholesterol, the liver also regulates glucose metabolism, makes proteins, and detoxifies the body, among other functions.

Obese patients often end up having really high total body cholesterol, such as high triglycerides, high LDL (the bad cholesterol) and low HDL (the good cholesterol). This is because, besides ingesting high cholesterol containing foods, their excess visceral or abdominal fat cells also secrete toxic substances that interfere with liver functions. Once the function of the liver is disrupted, everything it normally does goes haywire; that includes cholesterol homeostasis.

Triglycerides mostly come from animal fats and oils we eat, but they can also be converted from excess carbs and stored for later use. Too many triglycerides and LDL (bad cholesterol) promote fatty deposits along arteries, leading to development of atherosclerosis, heart disease, and stroke. This is because cholesterol plaques stimulate clot formation. The good cholesterol (HDL), on the other hand, encourages the removal of excess fatty deposits from blood vessels, thereby lowering the risk of aforementioned diseases.

Weight loss, diet changes, and exercise often improve cholesterol numbers. Note that some patients may have genetic reasons for their high cholesterol. These folks often require medication to achieve goal cholesterol levels even after making the appropriate lifestyle changes.

STROKE

Overweight individuals have a higher risk than their normal-weight counterparts of suffering from a stroke. Though strokes come in different forms, they mainly result from uncontrolled hypertension, untreated high cholesterol, or the combination.

We can't say that that *all* strokes are related to obesity, but it definitely contributes. There are two main types of stroke: ischemic and hemorrhagic. Ischemic strokes are caused by blockage of blood flow to the brain due to emboli (traveling blood clot) or thrombi (stationary blood clot). If you recall, we mentioned in earlier chapters that fat cells secrete substances that promote blood clotting, while high cholesterol deposits plaques that also stimulate clotting. This is a double whammy.

Hemorrhagic strokes, on the other hand, are caused by breakage or blowout of a weakened blood vessel wall in the brain, usually stemming from longstanding untreated hypertension.

Depending on what part of the brain is affected during a stroke, its physical effects can vary widely. For example, we can see trouble speaking, loss of balance and coordination, vision loss or blindness, trouble swallowing or hearing, memory loss, paralysis, and even breathing problems leading to need for life support. Essentially, stroke can rob you of the most basic abilities, leading to loss of your independence. The chances of having a stroke decrease as risk factors are removed.

DIABETES

Diabetes is a bit more complex than high blood pressure because there are so many regulatory systems involved in controlling the blood sugar. Obesity-related diabetes is essentially type 2 diabetes, which is a condition where there is resistance to the insulin secreted by the pancreas. This is different from type 1 diabetes, where the pancreas can't make any insulin. Insulin is one of the main hormones in the body that controls the cells' ability to take in and use glucose.

Up to 80 percent of people who are diagnosed with type 2 diabetes are obese, leading us to believe that the excess fat cells must be playing a role. Recent research findings from Harvard University, University of Pennsylvania, and Albert Einstein College of Medicine suggest that fat cells secrete hormones such as adiponectin and resistin that affect how sensitive certain cells and tissues are to the body's insulin, many times leading to resistance.

So, if the pancreas is producing insulin, but the fat cells are secreting hormones that resist it, that means there's excess glucose floating around in your system. Sooner or later, that can cause major devastations. Many times, diabetes is associated with nerve damage (pain, tingling, numbness in the hands and legs); eye damage (blindness); heart conditions (heart attacks); blood vessel damage (leading to need for amputations); and kidney damage (leaky kidney, spilling of protein in the urine, and need for dialysis).

Blood sugar numbers and insulin resistance usually improve with weight loss, but some damage caused by diabetes cannot be reversed once it's done. For example, blindness, amputations, kidney failure, and nerve pain do not go away with better numbers. In this instance, prevention is a lot better than cure!

HEART DISEASE

Heart disease is one of the major killers of an obese patient, who is up to 10 times more likely to be diagnosed with this condition. Many factors are considered when diagnosing heart disease. The first one is called atherosclerosis, or hardening of the arteries. Over time, calcium builds up on fatty deposits along the arteries, making the arteries tough and diminishing their normal function. The vessels become so hardened that the blood does not flow the way it's supposed to, and patients begin having symptoms such as chest pain, shortness of breath, and pain in the limbs thanks to lack of oxygen to tissues, organs, and the limbs.

Angina and myocardial infarction (heart attack) are results of diminished blood flow to the heart due to narrowing of the coronary arteries, which supply blood to the heart. Cholesterol deposits, high blood pressure, and diabetes all contribute to this problem. Excess fat cells in obese patients make matters worse by releasing substances that ramp up inflammation and fuel blood clotting. The result? When your physical activity increases even slightly—including just walking—blood can't flow fast enough through the narrowed space to supply the demand, thereby causing ischemia or death of the tissue from lack of oxygen. This is the chest pain you hear about leading up to a heart attack! Not good.

MUSCULOSKELETAL PROBLEMS

A lot of obese patients end up in doctors' offices for musculoskeletal problems such as lower back pain and knee joint pain. Many times, they are not aware that they already have heart disease, high blood pressure, or diabetes, either because they don't have any symptoms or they blame something else for them. For example, someone with angina, or chest pain, might think it's just heartburn. But a patient definitely recognizes unexplained back, knee, ankle, or hip pain. When a patient tells me she's having back pain and her BMI is well over 30, it's clear to me that the weight problem may be the cause of her pain or, at the very least, contributing to it. This is easy for anyone to understand; if you put an extra 100 pounds on a body that was designed to hold 150 pounds, musculoskeletal problems are inevitable.

Mechanically, most people's joints are not designed to carry 250+ pounds. The amount of lubrication, or "shock absorber," between the joints is only designed to carry the ideal body weight for that specific height, give or take a few pounds. When you have excess weight, the cartilage becomes worn early and the synovial fluid cushioning the joints gets pushed out of the way, leaving bone to rub on bone. How is it possible to start a fire by rubbing two sticks together? Friction and heat. The same effect happens when bone rubs on bone, only instead of fire, you get inflammation, swelling, redness, and pain (as seen in osteoarthritis). This can go on for years and, if it remains

The World Health Organization reports that osteoarthritis is one of the top leading causes of disability in men and women. unchecked, can destroy the joint entirely, leading to the need for knee replacement, hip replacement, or back surgery for compressed or herniated discs. The World Health Organization reports that osteoarthritis is one of the top leading causes of disability in men and women.

It has been estimated in multiple studies published in the *Journal of Rheumatology* that for every extra two pounds you gain, your risk of developing osteoarthritis increases by 10 percent. Even though a normal-weight person might also develop this condition later in life—after all, what else could you use daily for 80 years without it showing a little wear and tear?—it's common for obese people to suffer with it at an earlier age, such as in their 30s and 40s.

For the most part, patients agree with me when I tell them their weight is to blame for their musculoskeletal issues. A good number already know it is time to do something about their weight, but the question is whether it's too late for the joints. This is not a condition that is easily reversible once the weight is lost; once the damage is done, it's done.

Of course, for some, musculoskeletal problem and weight gain can be a vicious cycle. For example, obese patients with back or knee pain might start exercising to lose weight but find they can't exercise intensely enough to see encouraging results because of their pain. As they try harder, the pain flares up more, forcing them to back off and become inactive again. Result? Well, further weight gain. The most important thing here is not to lose hope but to keep working with your doctor, nutritionist, or trainer until you find a program that can work for you despite your limitations. Giving up could affect your mobility and independence for years to come. Never ideal.

RESPIRATORY PROBLEMS

Sleep apnea is a very well defined health risk of obesity. Mechanically, when a patient with excess weight lies down to sleep, all the extra tissue at the back of the throat relaxes and obstructs their airway. A neck size greater than 17 inches highly increases the risk, though thin people can also have sleep apnea. Naturally, this means they're not supplying enough oxygen to the brain, lungs, or the other organs in the body during these times of airway narrowing and obstruction. These patients might wake up gagging to reopen their airway because their brain senses the problem and screams, "Hey! I'm not getting enough oxygen here!" So they wake up briefly and then fall asleep again, only to reawaken this way 5 to 30 times per hour throughout the night. The periods are so brief that patients often don't remember having them, but their partners might complain about the loud snoring or periods where they stop breathing (the "apnea" in "sleep apnea"), followed by rough awakenings. By this point, many couples are sleeping in separate beds or separate rooms! The patients often report daytime sleepiness and exhaustion despite having "slept" for eight hours per night.

This is a lot of abuse for the body to take every night, and your partner's complaints may be the least of your worries. It's possible you'll start to develop hypertension, heart problems, memory problems, morning headaches, mood swings or feelings of depression, impotence, and even pulmonary hypertension, which is when pressure in the lungs increases to try to compensate for the lack of oxygen but ends up causing the right side of the heart to fail. This isn't good for your brain, lungs, or heart. Ever become breathless after walking for just a few minutes? Some patients will tell me, "I can't even make it up that one flight of stairs without stopping in the middle," or, "If I try to exert myself even a little bit with exercise, I'll die. I have to stop because I am out of breath." You might also be experiencing sleep apnea.

A syndrome that is very similar and often co-exists with sleep apnea is what we call obesity hypoventilation syndrome (OHS), also known as Pickwickian syndrome. It occurs only in morbidly obese people; that is, those with a BMI well over 40. OHS happens when you can't breathe deeply or rapidly enough for proper gas exchange to occur in the lungs, so the lungs don't get rid of all the carbon dioxide with each breath. Therefore, patients with OHS are different from those with simple obstructive sleep apnea because they have abnormally elevated carbon dioxide levels in their blood, even during the day when they shouldn't.

The treatment is the same for both conditions; both types of patients have to wear a facemask and use a machine called CPAP in bed at night to force air into their lungs. Tracheotomy surgery (creating an opening through the neck into the windpipe for breathing) is sometimes necessary for Pickwickian patients. Weight loss, however, is the ultimate cure.

INCREASED RISKS FOR CANCER

In the last decade, a lot of research findings support the notion that obesity increases your risk of certain cancers. We now know that certain types of cancers—such as breast, colon, endometrial, ovarian, esophageal, pancreatic, and prostate cancer—are found more in obese patients. The National Cancer Institute at the National Institutes of Health reported on cancer.gov that in 2002, about 41,000 new cases of cancer in the United States were estimated to be due to obesity. This means that about 3.2 percent of all new cancers are linked to obesity. It also estimated that, in the United States, 14 percent of deaths from cancer in men and 20 percent of deaths in women were due to being overweight or obese. These figures are even more grim now, as obesity rates have continued rising.

In November 2009, researchers with the American Institute for Cancer reported that more than 100,000 cases of cancer each year are caused by excess body fat. Specifically, 49 percent of endometrial cancer, 35 percent of esophageal cancer, 28 percent of pancreatic cancer, 24 percent of kidney cancer, 21 percent of gallbladder cancer, 17 percent of breast cancer, and 9 percent of colorectal cancer cases are associated with obesity.

Why do obese patients have an added risk? Experts aren't sure why extra fat leads to malignancies, but we do know that fat cells secrete substances such as hormones (estrogen, insulin, insulin-like growth factor, etc.) that can promote tumor growth. Fat cells also secrete compounds that increase blood vessel development, which cancer cells need for rapid growth and survival.

Fat cells put the body in a state of chronic inflammation by secreting inflammatory substances. Cancers recruit these substances to keep the immune system busy fighting unimportant problems while it has the space and time to invade and take over.

SYNDROME X

Metabolic Syndrome X is a fancy, crazy name given to a group of risk factors that could contribute to other diseases we've already discussed, such as coronary artery disease, stroke, and type 2 diabetes. A person with three or more of the following has this syndrome:

- Waist circumference greater that 40 inches in men; greater that 35 inches in women
- A serum triglyceride level above 150
- HDL cholesterol below 40 in men; below 50 in women
- Blood pressure above 135/85 or taking a hypertensive medication
- Fasting blood glucose above 110 or taking antidiabetic medication

One major risk factor is having a large amount of visceral fat—the so-called "middle age spread"—since these specialized fat cells secrete substances that promote *other* risks factors.

This is a huge problem! Once I measure my patients' visceral fat and find it too high, I tell them that their risk for heart attack and diabetes just doubled. It doesn't matter how much you weigh—having that much visceral fat is a risk factor on its own, separate from the generalized fat everywhere else.

The easiest tool I use to measure body fat is a body composition scale. Ranging in price from $50 and upward, you can find these scales at many online retailers, including Amazon, and departmental stores such as Walmart. The scale can tell you how much fat is in every segment of your body, including visceral fat. It works by sending weak electrical signals through your body when you step barefooted on the scale. Water—found in your muscle, tissue, blood, and bone—conducts the signal easily. Fat doesn't. So the speed of electrode return to the scale gives a clear understanding of the amount and types of tissues in your body. I highly recommend making the investment in a body composition scale, as it also often measures BMI and calculates your BMR.

Another way to quickly estimate your visceral fat is to measure your waist circumference. Again, greater than 40 inches in men and 35 inches in women is too high.

GYNECOLOGIC PROBLEMS

If you're an overweight woman, you may have experienced gynecologic problems such as abnormal periods and menstrual cycles. You might be flowing too much, too little, or irregularly. Infertility problems and other pregnancy complications are also very common. Obese women may end up having babies with high birth weight and are more likely to undergo a cesarean section. Of course, with a cesarean section in an obese person, there's additional risk with surgery thanks to breathing and anesthesia complications. Obese women are also at higher risk of death for their babies and themselves. And a lot of obese mothers develop gestational diabetes while pregnant.

If you're an overweight man, sorry, you are not excluded. You may be contending with impotence, low sperm count, gynecomastia (breast development), and decreased libido (low sex drive).

GALLBLADDER DISEASE

Obese individuals often have gallbladder problems and end up having their gallbladders surgically removed. The gallbladder normally stores bile, which is made by the liver to digest the fat in the food we eat. The liver, seeing a huge amount of fat constantly in the diet, continues to make more and more. After a while, stones start to form in the gallbladder, causing excruciating pain every time the gallbladder contracts or a stone moves.

Acid reflux is another disorder commonly seen in the obese. The acid reflux is caused when excess weight in the abdomen pushes up on the stomach and causes stomach acid to also get pushed up, reaching and irritating the esophagus (food pipe). The esophagus wall was never designed to see or tolerate acid, so it causes a pain we commonly call heartburn. Essentially, the acid is eating away at the esophagus. This can lead to ulcers, increased risk of perforation, bleeding, and eventually cancer if not treated or corrected promptly through lifestyle changes and weight loss.

NONALCOHOLIC STEATOHEPATITIS (NASH)

NASH, commonly called "fatty liver," is a condition in which there is excess fat stored in the liver. I see patients with that problem all the time. They come to me for a physical exam or general checkup, and after running routine labs, I find that their liver test numbers are abnormally elevated. In an obese person, NASH is high on my list of culprits, but I first have to rule out other causes such as infections (particularly viral hepatitis) and other conditions that can cause the elevation. When those tests come back negative, I usually get an ultrasound of the liver to confirm my initial suspicion. Fatty liver can occur without symptoms and is often called the "silent liver disease," but in the long term, it can cause irreversible scarring of the liver called cirrhosis. Fatty liver does improve with weight loss.

INCONTINENCE

No one likes talking about incontinence. We associate it with children and the elderly, people who have no control over their bodily functions. This adds insult to injury for the obese woman already suffering from body image issues. She might find herself leaking urine every time she coughs, laughs, or sneezes. The problem is caused by excess tissue in the abdominal area that pushes down on the bladder, just as in a pregnant woman whose incontinence stems from pressure from the baby. Part of the problem is that the sphincter muscles that should keep the urethra closed are also weakened, causing the woman to leak a bit with any added pressure.

There are other causes of urinary incontinence, but—as with anything else—we have to examine the patient's medical history thoroughly. A woman who has had a lot of babies might have urinary incontinence because the pelvic muscles have been stretched over the years from pregnancy and delivery. But many obese women already suffer with infertility and have not yet had any children, and certainly *not* many, so this is not the explanation for their incontinence. The good news? You guessed it. Once the patient loses weight, the problem typically goes away.

IMMUNE DEFICIENCIES

Do you catch cold more often than other people you know? Does it last longer? Do your wounds take a while to heal? It could be because your weight is affecting your immune system.

What happens is that fat cells secrete inflammatory substances into the bloodstream, interfering with immune system function and causing it to deal with diseases less efficiently than it would in most people. This is another reason why obese patients' risk of surgery is usually higher than most—they don't heal as well and have greater risks of complications because their immune system is preoccupied with other things, instead of fighting infection and helping with wound healing.

PSYCHOSOCIAL EFFECTS

Despite how serious all the physical effects of excess weight are, psychosocial effects are sometimes the most damaging. I often see patients who are socially isolated, intimidated, and bullied. They may be viewed as lazy, as if they don't have willpower to do something about their condition. A lot of obese people can't or don't have romantic relationships because of low self-esteem, and others are discriminated against at work, where hiring managers may see them as "undesirable" employees. In the face of all this, it's almost impossible to fight the depression that comes along. Many of my patients would rather just be alone, where there is no fear of being taunted. I often refer to this depression as "Tears of Obesity." (And, hey, I've been there!) On average, at least one patient a day will cry Tears of Obesity. They'll tell me, "I already know I have diabetes, high blood pressure, and joint problems. What else now?" I usually end up having to diagnose them with yet another obesity-related condition, forcing them to confront the reality that their condition is killing them, even though they feel they are doing everything they can. Some patients feel limited by their condition and will tell me, "I can't move because my back hurts," or, "I want to lose this weight, and I am watching what I eat, but I am really hungry all the time." I hear, "I have cut out fatty foods," and, "I've started baking everything, eating more veggies, even started walking, but I'm not losing anything," and they end up crying more. Tears of Obesity.

Many of my obese patients feel helpless. I had a man who came in upset as he realized the effects that obesity was having on his life. His daughter had just had a baby, and now he was a grandfather, worrying that he would not be around to see his grandchildren grow up. Tears of Obesity.

A 34-year-old female patient confessed her worry that, with all the extra weight she is carrying, she will never meet someone to spend her life with, never be able to have a baby because of difficulty getting pregnant. She cried in my office, too.

Another patient, a 50-year-old male and former body builder, suffered a back injury in a motorbike accident. As a result, over the course of six months or so, he gained some weight. After his back injury had healed, he tried to go back to his routine at the gym, but his back acted up every time. Because he couldn't exercise anymore, he slowly started gaining more weight. Eventually, he got to the point where he was having trouble walking around. On top of the weight struggle, he had recently lost his dad. He said that his dad had been in a state where they'd had to do everything for him—clean him, bathe him, feed him—and my patient saw himself heading in that direction. He was considering a gastric bypass surgery when I met him, and I could immediately tell he was depressed. He couldn't even raise his head to look at me as he told me about everything he'd been through.

Fortunately, this patient was willing to try a pretty unconventional weight loss method—the same one that helped me. His eyes lit up as I explained it, and I could see that this was the hope he needed to pull him out of his depression. In just one week on the program, he lost eight pounds. That weight loss alone was enough to lower his blood glucose levels from 250 to 176. I cut his insulin dose in half. That is a prime example of how, when you start losing the weight, all those crazy substances secreted by fat cells start to slow down! He is hopeful that he can be off insulin in no time if he continues to lose weight on this program.

Like him, you *can* and *will* see improved health and decreased symptoms of other conditions once you begin managing your weight in an effective way. And that is what I am here to help you do.

PART II

WHAT ARE MY OPTIONS?

CHAPTER 5

EAT **LESS**, EXERCISE **MORE**— **OR**...

IF you've identified yourself as among the group that is eating too much or eating all the wrong foods and, ahem, *lacking* in the exercise department, congratulations. In recognizing this as the problem, you've just done half the work to reach your goals.

Now what?

THE OTHER HALF OF THE WORK

Some people say diets don't work. Others say diets work and it's *people* who don't. Me? I'm kind of in the middle, because I believe diets work *if*, and only if, you can stick to them.

So what makes you stick to them?

Well, most diets are designed around a low caloric intake— they have reduced the amount of calories that you're going to take in, while still trying to provide your body with most of the essential nutrients you need. Occasionally, you'll find a diet that completely eliminates a food group, but most try to maintain nutritional requirements. Among all the numerous options out there, you *must* find a diet that fits into your lifestyle. Otherwise, it won't work for you in the long run.

I had a patient recently to whom I was explaining some weight loss options. When I showed him the diet he had to be on, he told me he doesn't, and wouldn't, eat vegetables. That means that particular diet would not work for him, no matter how effective, because it *required* eating plenty of vegetables. If he hadn't admitted that, I would have sent him on his way thinking that he was going to stick to the diet when, in reality, he would not. He might try it for a few days, maybe even a couple of weeks, but in the end, he would abandon it because it wasn't the right fit for him. I can't force him to eat what he doesn't want to; he is a grown man, a *big* man, for that matter. I can only advise him that it would be healthy for him to start adding vegetables to his meals.

At that point with a patient, it's time to look at other diet options. As far as I'm concerned, a diet plan *must* be acceptable to the patient in order to sustain it for a long time. The key principle behind a good diet is that it should *improve* your health and happiness, not impair them.

Most people who stay on diets for a long time tell me it helps to have what they call a "free day." That is, they adhere strictly to the diet six days out of the week and have one day to look forward to eating whatever they want. Patients who prefer these diets say that the free day motivates them to get through the other six days. To me, any diet that incorporates a free day that *won't* undo the benefits of the first six is probably a great choice.

Aside from any particular diet (which I'll soon cover), you should look at your food in terms of **quantity control** and **quality control**. If you're eating too much, the solution becomes portion control. If your "too much" boils down to the *quality* of your food, we must discuss nutritional value. By understanding both and following some simple guidelines, it's possible to live free from any formal "diet."

QUANTITY CONTROL

Let's get something straight: you do *not* have to count every calorie you eat. Who has time for that? Unless you're like me and know exactly how many calories are in every single food item (I've done my research!), accurate calorie counting is frustrating and time-consuming. Instead, follow these tips for estimating portions and calories.

One serving of **protein** should not be bigger than the palm of your hand, or around the size of a deck of cards. A portion this size is around 100 calories, if it's lean.

If you're going to eat **carbs**, such as rice or potatoes, your portion shouldn't be bigger than a clenched fist.

Whatever amount of steamed or raw **vegetables** you can fit in a cupped palm is a good portion for each meal. But there's leeway here! Want more broccoli? Go for it.

Nuts make a great midday snack, but go small. A correct portion is the size of a golf ball.

If you eat three balanced meals a day with these portions, you can scratch calorie counting off your to-do list.

QUANTITY CONTROL TIPS AND TRICKS

- Put your food in the center of your plate. When it is centered, rather than overflowing off the sides of your plate, you will *see* that the quantity is enough to fill you. Your stomach is only about the size of your fist. Shocking? I know. It's hard to believe only because many of us have worked hard over the years to stretch and over-stretch our stomachs so they are now able to hold a lot more food. We need it to bounce back to its ideal size.

- If you can eat frequently during the day, it will keep you from overdoing it during your three main meals. I encourage my patients to have a snack mid-morning, another mid-afternoon, and one right before dinner or shortly after. However, these snacks should be **healthy**—shoot for fruits, nuts, and crunchy veggies—not what you find in most workplace vending machines or break rooms.

- Don't wait until you're very hungry to start eating. Waiting causes you to overestimate how much you should eat, because you're measuring based on your current appetite. If you eat before your hunger gets out of hand, you can more easily stick to reasonable portions. It's the same principle used when people say, "Don't go grocery shopping on an empty stomach." You'd buy everything and anything.

- If you're eating out, split an entree with a friend or get a to-go box and split the meal in half before you start eating. Restaurants portion sizes are two to three times larger than you need, so once you visually remove half from your plate, you can ignore it and eat the appropriate amount.

- Be aware of the calories in drinks. You may think you're just quenching your thirst, but a fancy coffee or large soda can contain upwards of 400 calories!

- Condiments and toppings are sneaky! Mayonnaise, opaque sauces and marinades, cheese, bacon, etc., are all loaded with fat and calories. We tend to forget that these add-ons contribute to what we've consumed in a day, but adding a few strips of bacon to a sandwich can throw an extra 100 calories onto your meal.

- Want to lose twice as much weight as you ordinarily might? Keep a food journal. It has been shown that dieters who write down everything they eat lose double the weight of their non-writing counterparts. And there's an app for that—for less than a buck, you can get a comprehensive tool by searching for "food diary" in your phone's app store or market place. There are many different options, but a free one I use is called dailyburn. It can help track your nutrition, exercises, and weight. Keep track *as* you eat, rather than after; you'll be more accurate that way.

QUALITY CONTROL

When focusing on quality, concentrate on eating healthy foods—as healthy as you can possibly eat.

Some people assume anything good for you must taste bad, but this is not true. What *is* true is that the "reward center" in our brains has been altered; because of the fast food industry, a lot of us have a hard time recognizing food in its natural state as "good tasting." If this is the case for you, fast food is probably irresistible, whereas the natural and healthy stuff just fills you up but doesn't make you say, "Yum!" It doesn't hit your reward center, so you don't find yourself saying, "Oh, God, I have to have that grapefruit again!" You must retrain your brain.

Start by reminding yourself that the natural state of food is what your body really needs. Your body is desperate for vitamins, nutrients, and fiber. Remember, where you are is likely the culmination of years of eating bad food. It's possible you've been feasting on reward center type foods as far back as childhood. When you were a kid and being good, your mom didn't offer you carrots or apples for a reward; she gave you a cookie or candy! Now you're grown up and being diagnosed with all these weight-related conditions, and your doctor is ordering you to eat fresh fruits, steamed vegetables … without cheese! It takes work to convince your taste buds to recognize and enjoy food that is good for you. But it *can* happen. Start by reminding yourself that the natural state of food is what your body really needs. Your body is desperate for vitamins, nutrients, and fiber. Talk yourself through it as often as you need; one day, you'll find that you no longer compare apples to French fries.

The problem with most diets is that they try to combat years of reward center wiring in just a few short days or weeks. It's unrealistic. Changes that will last need to be made more slowly. Don't go from a totally unhealthy diet with fried foods and soda drinking straight to "the raw food diet," for example. It's too much of a shock. Wean slowly.

So, as far as quality control *without* complicated rules goes, I tell my patients to eat:

- **Lean protein:** chicken breast without skin, turkey breast, lean steaks and ground beef (as close to 95 percent lean as possible), mostly egg whites instead of the whole egg (five egg whites equals the same amount of calories in one whole egg), and cottage cheese. These lean proteins provide the essential amino acids—or building blocks for muscles—enzymes, and antibodies the body needs.

- **Complex carbohydrates:** 100 percent wheat, whole grains, beans, and most vegetables. High fiber is necessary so it breaks down slowly and does not spike your blood sugar. Since all carbohydrates break down to glucose, we want to eat those that release slowly. If you eat carbs that release quickly, your sugar will spike, and then it will crash. We all know what happens then: "I'm *starving!*"

- **Vitamins and minerals:** Reach for fresh fruits and vegetables. The greener the leaf is, the more loaded with vitamins. Eat a variety of fruits, but be careful with really sweet ones. Bananas are good, for example, but not as good as apples because bananas have more sugar and carbs.

- **Essential fats:** olive oil, safflower oil, fish oil, canola oil, Omega 3 fatty acids, and Omega 6 (found in salmon, tuna) are what your body craves. A lot of people worry that eating essential fats and oils will make them fat, but it doesn't work that way. The reason they're called *essential* is because our cells need them to repair their membranes and as building blocks for other functions. Meanwhile, we have to consume them because our bodies cannot manufacture them. The types of fats you want to limit are the saturated fats and the trans fat, which you find in margarine, sweets, and fried foods.

- **Water:** I'm not going to tell you exactly how much water to drink because it varies by person. What I *will* say is to look at your urine. If it's clear, you're consuming a good amount of water. If it's yellow or dark, you need to drink more. Most people need between six to eight glasses of water (eight ounces per glass) per day. But the right amount for you is the amount that makes your urine almost clear.

Easy enough, right? It's about to get easier (sort of).

FOODS TO AVOID

Stay away from deep-fried foods, heavy sauces, thick creamy salad dressings (if you can't see through it, it's probably not good for you!), sugary foods, and stuffed anything (unless it's Thanksgiving!). And for God's sake, just say no to anything labeled "smothered," "battered," or "country style." Our reward center thinking tells us these terms are synonymous with "delicious," but they're direct barriers to your weight loss goals.

Soda is another offender. I recommend replacing your daily soda fix (or fixes) with carbonated mineral water. It fizzes just like your favorite soft drink, and you can switch it up by adding a sweetener like Stevia that comes in different flavors and still has zero calories. Stevia is from a natural leaf, not a chemical that was made in the lab.

Why not diet sodas? They use a lot of the artificial sugars, and when the tongue tastes them, the body gears up for the next step. Thinking it's about to receive *real* sugar, it releases insulin and other chemicals to break down the sugar only to find that it wasn't sugar at all. What happens? You get hungry! When I was in college, I tried drinking Diet Mountain Dew because I needed the caffeine and didn't want the calories. I found that roughly an hour later—every time—I was crazy hungry! I'd end up eating whatever was available in the school, usually vending machine chocolate candy bars or McDonald's chicken fingers or chicken nuggets, to ease that hunger. I would have been better off drinking regular Mountain Dew to start with. (But even *better* off with just plain coffee.)

THE CASE FOR EXERCISE

More exercise is good for you, but what we've found is that exercise by itself doesn't produce major weight loss. Yes, you're building muscle, and yes, muscle burns more calories and takes less room than fat because it's more compact. But you find yourself frustrated because the number on the scale isn't changing. And, as we all know, frustration is the precursor to, "Oh, I give up!" (Sound familiar?) The best thing to do is start an exercise routine at the same time as a diet.

Patients often ask me for guidelines about exercise. If you are 18 or over, you should be doing at least 150 minutes of moderate intensity exercise (like brisk walking, swimming, or dancing) per week. For added benefit, you should add two or more days per week of muscle strengthening or a core workout, such as pushups or sit-ups, for around 30 minutes each day.

If you are doing vigorous exercise, which burns even more calories—jogging, running, spinning—I recommend 75 minutes per week. You don't have to do it all in one or two sessions; break it down to several 15–30 minute sessions per week if that's easier to incorporate into your lifestyle. Studies have shown that you get the same effect this way as you would by doing fewer, longer workouts per week.

For children, one hour of aerobic activity, such as walking or running, three times a week is recommended for muscle strengthening. They should also do one hour of bone strengthening, such as jump rope, three times a week. Starting your children on exercise at an early age will help them develop good habits and maintain their health throughout their lives. Do not wait until they're overweight or obese teenagers. You can't make teenagers do anything, fat or thin.

FINDING THE RIGHT EXERCISE FOR YOU

When it comes to exercise, you have to find the right one for you. The "right one" is an activity *you* find fun (or at least more fun than others). Not everybody needs to go to the gym. Not everyone likes treadmills. And if you're doing something you don't like, you're not likely to stick to it long term. So if you like dancing, swimming, or jump roping, do those! For me, it was bike riding. I loved it because it was outdoors and I could observe the scenery around me. I was experiencing nature, the wind blowing through my hair, and I enjoyed the fresh air. It worked for me, and I looked forward to it! Find something you look forward to doing.

Even when you're doing something you like, you can get bored with the same routine every day. Change it up every now and then. Go with a friend to a yoga class, play catch, take a swim, or do something else every now and then to mix it up. Think about activities you enjoy, and see if you can work in a bit of exercise with them.

As always, check with your doctor before beginning any exercise program. Granted, I can tell you that when a patient informs me she wants to begin exercising, I say, "Please! Thank you!" But if you do have joint problems and other conditions, consulting with your doctor before you begin a routine will help you find activities that will do more good than damage to you and your body. I ended up working out on the elliptical instead of biking when my knees acted up because it was less strenuous on my joints; your doctor will be able to recommend what's best for your unique physical condition.

One exercise you can do regardless of how limited in mobility you are is water aerobics. Water aerobics is awesome because it isn't just low-impact exercise; it's *no*-impact. You're able to move that joint that was a little stiff, and you don't have gravity working against you. This is a great example of being able to find an exercise solution no matter what your limitations are.

FIND A WORKOUT BUDDY

Sometimes having a partner to motivate you can help on days you're feeling discouraged. A partner can push you and encourage you. Support is key in this process! My grandmother was my workout buddy when she visited me from Nigeria. After she returned home, I couldn't find anyone to work out with because of my crazy work schedule. So, what did I do? I paid my workout buddy … my trainer. Yours can be a lot cheaper; just ask your friends, coworkers, or neighbors. Most will be willing to support you, at least for a while, since they are looking for support themselves.

FEEL GOOD!

Another perk to exercise is the feel-good chemical our bodies release when we work out. Daily runners can tell you all about this. For them, a "day off" from running isn't a reward; they'll say they don't feel as good as the days they do run. That's because, on those days off, their bodies don't secrete endorphins, a chemical that infuses you with energy and gives you a good outlook on life. You get used to having that in your system when you exercise regularly. Some people will even tell you they feel tired during the day, but when they get to the gym and start working out, they feel better. It's all about the endorphins. Give it a shot!

NO EXCUSES

I've heard them all.

Your excuse: I don't have time.

My response: You make time for things that are important for you. You make time to eat, take the kids to school, work, clean the house, and the list goes on. If you prioritize your health, you will find the time for exercise. It might mean you need to wake up earlier or go to sleep later on those three days per week. But you make time.

Your excuse: I have joint pain.

My response: Remember water aerobics?

Your excuse: I'm self-conscious.

My response: Exercise does not have to be in a gym or with a trainer. Go outside and get a buddy or your partner to take a walk, hike, or bike ride with you.

What's your excuse? Get it to me and I'm sure we'll find a solution.

The point here is this: eating right and exercising doesn't have to be a maze full of trick corners and impossible boundaries. If you can stick to the basic guidelines in this chapter, you'll be well on your way to (re)discovering a healthier, happier you. Want to go a step further by defining a diet plan that will work? We'll do that, too. But, first, the reason many diets fail ...

CHAPTER 6

EMOTIONAL
EATING

EMOTIONAL eating is the enemy. You begin a diet and maybe do well the first week; you stick to the guidelines and possibly even drop a few pounds. It's hard work, but you feel a little hopeful. Then the second week, something triggers your emotions—a fight with a spouse, a bad review at work, a sick child—and, just like that, you fall off the wagon and cheat. Once you've done this, the guilt stays with you, and you try to suppress the guilty feelings with even more food. At that point, the diet is basically over.

Emotional eating is often used to deal with life's struggles. Instead of working on how to deal with anger, loneliness, self-doubt, frustration, or other emotions, we continue to cover up our feelings with food. Many times, we don't even know this is the reason our diets aren't working, because eating for comfort is something we have known since we were babies. Think about it—when you cried, your mother gave you some milk. When you fell and hurt yourself, your mother might have fixed you up and given you a little piece of candy to make you feel better. When you got a good grade on a test, you were taken out for ice cream after school. Food as comfort or reward is something we have grown accustomed to; it's no wonder diets are so difficult to maintain!

So how do you know that you are an emotional eater? Maybe you feel as if you have nothing to offer other people. Perhaps there is the feeling of anger because of a conflict with family members or loved ones, or you are experiencing friction with a colleague, boss, or friend. Maybe you are trying to accomplish something and are overwhelmed by the effort or frustrated by your lack of success . Maybe you feel as if you are not in charge of your own life. Maybe you are feeling empty because a relationship didn't work out or feeling lonely because you have no family members living close by. Any of these situations could trigger emotional eating habits, and recognizing the signs is the first step to addressing the problem.

PHANTOM HUNGER OR REAL HUNGER?

To uncover whether you're emotionally eating—and, if so, what your triggers are—you have to dig deep and do some self-examination. You have to investigate your habits and explore what is really going on. I had to go through this myself; I gained the weight because I was eating to stop the feelings of loneliness and sadness from my relationship breakup, as well as the stress of my residency training program. But in order to reach this diagnosis, I had to start evaluating where my hunger was coming from: was it coming from my stomach—real, physical hunger? Or was the hunger in my head?

Physical hunger comes on slowly—it is a growing sensation that starts because your stomach feels empty, and there are cues like stomach growling and cramping called hunger pangs. You'll notice the desire for food is not specific—you are not craving ice cream; you are just looking for something to fill your stomach.

Hunger in your head, or "phantom hunger," comes on suddenly, and it's *specific*. Phantom hunger would never be satisfied with broccoli. It wants comfort food. Phantom hunger causes you to eat quickly and continue eating even when you are full.

Once you can differentiate between physical hunger and phantom hunger, and you realize that phantom hunger is attacking you, you need to take a look at what emotion you are trying to stuff away or cover up. Maybe your boss just made you mad, or you ran into an ex, and suddenly all you can think about is chocolate. A patient once told me that when she was home alone, she had to constantly chew on something because she couldn't stand the quietness. She was eating to cover up her loneliness. Recognizing your triggers will give you the power to incorporate some of the following strategies for vanquishing phantom hunger.

DISTRACT YOURSELF

To my patient who couldn't stand the quiet, I asked, "Well, what other activities could you do to rid yourself of the loneliness?" I suggested that when she reaches that point of phantom hunger, she should go for a walk, call a friend, play with her pet, listen to music, or dance. The point is: distract yourself!

When I was overeating, I got into a routine of eating when I was not hungry. I would eat breakfast around 7:30 a.m. and be at work by 8:00. An hour later, I suddenly felt hungry again, so I went in search of the vending machines. I found myself eating a Snickers bar, thinking, *It's healthy— it has peanuts!* In reality, I wasn't hungry. I was looking for something to do. But why? What was my trigger?

Once I realized my hunger was of the phantom variety, I was able to change my behavior. Instead of my purposeful (and guilty) midmorning stride to the vending machines, I forced myself to work on reports and presentations. What I realized was that I was trying to avoid doing those reports by stuffing myself with a Snickers bar! It was my way of procrastinating. Once I recognized that, I could go about my day. It just required taking control of my thought process.

Now, I find that if I can stay away from eating whatever my phantom hunger wants for about 20 minutes, I often forget about it. Try it. Find something else to do to occupy your time during those sudden, fierce cravings. If you can avoid the temptation even 50 percent of the time, you're winning.

AVOID SKIPPING MEALS

Another way to deal with emotional eating is to avoid skipping meals and pack healthy snacks with you as often as you can. One of the things about skipping meals is that you end up building a bigger appetite for later. For example, sometimes I get too busy at work to eat lunch. By the time I leave, I'm super hungry and all I can see on my drive home are billboards for fast food places. Maybe I'm able to resist pulling into a drive-thru, but I'm already thinking about the refrigerator and what I will eat when I get home.

Before I even change out of my work clothes, I'm raiding the fridge. Of course, the first thing I grab is the heavy stuff—I'm hungry! Why would I go for the carrots?—and you know I'm going to eat standing up. After all, it doesn't count as real food or a *meal* if you're standing up, right? So now dinner comes around, and my appetite's only been whetted. Bring on the larger-than-usual portion size. Twenty minutes later, I'm stuffed and kicking myself. *I just blew my diet again!* From there, the vicious cycle continues. My self-worth is down the drain, and guess what I'm going to do to stop that flood of emotions? I'm going to grab some popcorn and sit down to watch some television. My suggestion? Don't skip meals!

DO NOT DEPRIVE YOURSELF

We should also try not to completely deprive ourselves of certain foods. That feeling of deprivation increases the reward value of the food, especially when you're an emotional eater. You may think you're absolutely not allowed to have any carbs or sugar or whatever is restricted on a particular diet, and all of a sudden the phantom hunger comes on and that forbidden fruit is exactly what you are going to want. My suggestion? Decide ahead of time when to reward yourself with foods that fall in this category for you. Also decide how much of it to eat. For example, I love popsicles. I know they're full of sugar, so I try to limit my intake. But I decided to eat them at my friend's house, who buys them occasionally for his kids. Since the popsicles belong to the kids, I'm able to limit myself to just one per visit!

MANAGE STRESS

To handle emotional eating, you have to learn how to manage stress. A patient I recently started on a program has a huge amount of stress from home and work. She is the sole caregiver of a husband who is disabled from two strokes and a mother whose multiple medical problems take her in and out of the hospital. On top of that, my patient has several medical problems herself on top of be-ing obese—*and* her work is stressful. She broke down and said, "I can't stay on this diet—it's not that it's not working; it's just that I need an outlet for my stress, and food is one of the only places I can go."

As a doctor, I know that putting a patient on a diet to try to help her lose weight without managing the stress in her life is not going to work. As I told her, "Even if you get the weight off, you are going to put it right back on, because you're going to go back into the same stressful environment." So we decided to put the diet aside. Now what we've done is find ways to relieve her stress at home by hiring help. This has freed up some time for her to deal better with the stress at work. She has already started los-ing some weight on her own even without a formal diet. This is most likely because her cortisol (stress hormone) level went down significantly.

What are your stressors? Write them down. It's important to find an outlet or outlets to relieve the stress in your life. If you need help around the house, maybe assigning chore lists to your family or adjusting your budget to afford biweekly housekeeping would help. Maybe yoga or deep breathing and meditation can help manage the stress from work. Maybe your religious beliefs or faith will calm your mind. Whatever it is, you need to find a personal outlet.

LEARN TO FORGIVE YOURSELF
You have to learn to forgive yourself when you do slip up. For example, if I have eaten that Snickers bar at work to put off doing my reports, I need to recognize that one mistake is not going to make me gain 10 pounds. If I cor-rect my behavior, I can keep myself on track for the rest

of the day, rather than berate myself for "ruining my diet." Once emotional eaters go down that road of self-doubt and self-worthlessness, we tend to spiral into a vicious cycle that brings us back to eating more and more. You have to cut yourself some slack. Realize that tomorrow is another day. For that matter, today isn't over yet; you can still make decisions that will make you feel good about yourself the rest of the time.

GET HELP WHEN YOU NEED IT

If you are an emotional eater suffering from depression, anxiety, or feelings of emptiness or loneliness, you need to seek help. Cognitive behavioral therapy is what a lot of therapists use to treat people who are emotional eaters. The goal is to dig deeply into what is causing you to have those feelings. Then you are taught how to deal with those emotions directly so as not to jeopardize your weight loss efforts—or other life goals, for that matter.

Though I (misguidedly) chose not to see a therapist, I realized that my behavior was not ordinary and I could not deal with it on my own. I needed to find answers, so I checked out book after book and read article after article on emotional eating. One book I found especially helpful was *Shrink Yourself: Break Free From Emotional Eating Forever*, by Dr. Roger Gould. It really helped me with my self-investigation about this disorder.

Another option is a program called Overeaters Anonymous (OA). Similar to Alcoholics Anonymous and Narcotics Anonymous, this program teaches its members 12 steps to overcoming their addiction to food. OA's 12 steps are each associated with a spiritual principal:

1 **Honesty:** we admitted we were powerless over food—that our lives had become unmanageable.

2 **Hope:** came to believe that a Power greater than ourselves could restore us to sanity.

3 **Faith:** made a decision to turn our will and our lives over to the care of God as we understood Him.

4 **Courage:** made a searching and fearless moral inventory of ourselves.

5 **Integrity:** admitted to God, to ourselves, and to another human being the exact nature of our wrongs.

6 **Willingness:** were entirely ready to have God remove all these defects of character.

7 **Humility:** humbly asked Him to remove our shortcomings.

8 **Self-discipline:** made a list of all persons we had harmed and became willing to make amends to them all.

9 **Love for others:** made direct amends to such people wherever possible, except when to do so would injure them or others.

10 **Perseverance:** continued to take personal inventory and, when we were wrong, promptly admitted it.

11 **Spiritual awareness:** sought through prayer and meditation to improve our conscious contact with God as we understood Him, praying only for knowledge of His will for us and the power to carry that out.

12 **Service:** having had a spiritual awakening as the result of these Steps, we tried to carry this message to compulsive overeaters and to practice these principles in all our affairs.[1]

---

1 Permission to use the Twelve Steps of Alcoholics Anonymous for adaptation granted by AA World Services, Inc.

Whatever road you choose to help overcome emotional eating, *choose* one. Put your reasons aside and seek help. If I had followed my own advice, I probably would have gotten out of the depression sooner and saved myself another 10–15 pounds of weight gain. I also might have found more success sooner using one of the diets in the next chapter.

CHAPTER 7

DIETS 101

NOT all diets are created equal. You have to find a plan that will work for you. I tried what seemed like dozens throughout my weight loss journey. And if I haven't tried one, my patients have, and I've read all about them! Let me fill you in.

THE 3-HOUR DIET

Designed by Jorge Cruise, who is a diet coach/fitness journalist, the 3-Hour Diet is based on the notion that eating every three hours will stabilize your blood sugar and reduce your levels of cortisol, a stress hormone that contributes to weight gain. The premise is that because you are eating as opposed to dieting, you will be able to stick to this program and lose weight—at a rate of 8–10 pounds per month. Not bad.

For me, the problem with this diet was that it didn't restrict any food groups. It didn't ask you to limit your carbs, nor did it encourage calorie counting. Cruise just said to be wise and split your meals into six separate portions, eating every three hours with your last meal three hours before bed. His theory was that because your metabolism would be boosted by frequent eating, you would burn extra calories and lose weight.

That's all well and good; everybody can eat every three hours if you allow them to! But for people who already have trouble with portion control, designating six different times to sit at a table and eat is a recipe (pardon the pun) for overeating every time. I learned this firsthand when I tried it.

The 3-Hour Diet is based on the notion that eating every three hours will stabilize your blood sugar and reduce your levels of cortisol, a stress hormone that contributes to weight gain.

I would start well with breakfast, do maybe just some egg whites and toast, and go about my day. At work, roughly around ten or eleven a.m., I would have to eat a snack. Now, unless I planned way ahead to bring healthy snacks to work, my snack ended up being something from the cafeteria or the vending machines. Probably not exactly what Cruise had in mind. Then, a short while later, I ate lunch. I was supposed to limit my meal to around 400 calories, but that didn't happen. I ate the same size lunch that I had always eaten, and then three hours later, I would go snack because I was allowed—no, *encouraged!* Now, it might have been a healthy snack on the days I planned ahead, but the reality was that I wasn't even hungry—which, of course, didn't make me limit the size of my dinner later. I ate as I normally would, with another snack before bed for good measure.

My results: I was on this diet for two weeks, and do I really need to tell you I didn't lose weight? I knew it was my fault for not cutting down my portion sizes (and, thus, calories), but this is the problem I see with anyone else who has tried this diet. It's simply counterintuitive for someone who already has issues with limiting portion size. However, for more detailed information on the 3-Hour Diet, visit www.3hourdiet.com.

THE ATKINS DIET

As most people know, the Atkins Diet is one of the most popular diets out there and is based on removing carbs from your food plane. Dr. Robert C. Atkins believes that limiting carbs to a great degree helps in losing weight and maintaining a healthy weight.

The diet is broken into four stages. In Phase 1, or the Induction, you're allowed only 20 grams of carbs (that's almost nothing: six cups of salad or two cups of a low-carb veggie) per day. The idea is that you can lose up to 15 pounds in these first two weeks, jumpstarting your diet. In Phase 2, or Ongoing Weight Loss, you begin reintroducing *some* carbs back into your diet; you add five more grams of carbs per week in this phase. You still continue to lose weight, the diets says, just a little more slowly. Then comes Phase 3, the Pre-Maintenance. By now, you're supposed to be fairly close to your goal (say, 10 pounds off), and you start to increase the amounts of fruits and vegetables you eat so that you add another 10 grams of carbs per week to your diet. In Phase 4, Lifetime Maintenance, you should have reached your goal and know which foods to eat and which to stay away from—essentially, pure carbs such as bread and potatoes. Most dieters fall between 50–100 grams of carbs per day when they are done.

My issue with this diet is there are no restrictions on how much or what kinds of *protein* to stick to. The diet doesn't say lean protein, so fatty, oily foods like yolk, sausage, and bacon are totally permissible. This is a little worrisome to me because you are consuming unsaturated fats and trans fats, all of which can have devastating effects on your arteries—and the diet doesn't really encourage exercise, either. This raises a concern about the cardiac health of people doing this diet, many of whom *already* have increased risk of heart disease.

Another potential problem is the possibility of this diet affecting people's brain health and mental clarity. When your body is breaking down mainly proteins and fats for energy, it builds up ketones, which replace glucose in the brain for energy. This can sometimes create a sense of "fogginess," which many patients on this diet report, especially in the first week of their induction phase. This may partly be due to the fact that you are also not eating the brain's favorite food, which is pure glucose. Many patients who stick to the diet eventually make it past this phase but report not being themselves during those "foggy" times.

That all said, this diet works for a lot of people. They lose a significant amount of weight and swear by Atkins. I think the reason it works is partly due to calorie reduction as well as carb reduction. Quite simply, you get sick of eating oily, fatty foods all the time. By not eating carbs and eating more protein and fatty foods, you get fuller for longer periods of time. So you end up not eating as much as you used to—not because you're intentionally cutting calories but because you're tired of the foods you're allowed to eat.

My results: I tried it and ate only protein and fats for the first two weeks. I lasted only another week into the second phase before I had to quit. I lost about two, maybe three, pounds the entire time I was on the diet. And I just kept thinking about what my next meal was going to be. I'd look at my lunch and think, *If I eat this turkey sandwich, I can only have the meat, so what else am I going to eat to make me feel full?* I was constantly thinking in terms of my diet, and that just didn't work for me.

Then there was the "forbidden fruit" element. When you are prohibited from a certain food group, like carbs, you crave those things even more. I could not stop thinking about eating something else other than this fatty protein. Every time I saw bread, I desperately wanted a slice. Though I can't say I felt "foggy," I couldn't see myself being on this diet for a lifetime. But you may have different results. For more detailed information on the Atkins diet, visit www.atkins.com.

THE SOUTH BEACH DIET

The South Beach Diet was designed by Dr. Arthur Agatston, a preventative cardiologist, and his ideas are very similar to the principles of the Atkins diet. When Dr. Agatston saw all the complaints regarding the Atkins diet and how it could lead to heart problems, he created the South Beach Diet to be a healthier version. This diet eliminates all the bad fatty proteins that the Atkins diet allows you to eat, and he added low glycemic vegetables to the program. So, while you can't have, say, potatoes on South Beach, you *can* eat whole grains and fruits that are high in fiber and grains without too many carbs.

The South Beach Diet runs in three phases. Phase 1 lasts for two weeks and is geared to help you lose cravings for sugars and refined starches. In Phase 2, you start to introduce more low glycemic veggies and fruits and some good carbs. This phase is where you're supposed to lose most of your weight, and it is where Dr. Agatston recommends you start if you have less than 10 pounds to lose. Finally, there is Phase 3, or the lifetime maintenance phase, where the dieter is not given a list of prohibited foods but rather expected to simply live by the principles of this diet learned in the other phases.

My results: After the first phase, the diet claims your cravings will be curbed. Not so for me. I still craved carbs! (Forbidden fruit.) I lasted about two weeks into the second phase of this diet, losing around a pound a week, but fell off the wagon again. First, the diet allows snacking, which I liked, but that is where I started to blow it. If I packed my own snacks, I was fine; if I forgot and started getting hungry, however, I didn't always make the best choices.

In all, there was so much meal planning involved that it didn't fit into my hectic schedule. I needed a diet that was simpler. There were also no exercise recommendations in the original program. Over time, though, the diet has evolved with popularity and now has added exercise to its newest revolution guidelines. For more detailed information on the South Beach Diet, go to www.southbeachdiet. com.

JENNY CRAIG WEIGHT LOSS PROGRAM

I guarantee you have seen these commercials on TV. The Jenny Craig diet program works by helping you eat already prepared prepackaged foods that you order as part of the program. It also includes weekly weigh-ins, during which you attend a motivational session with your weight loss counselor. Does this system work? Yes. You don't have to think about what you are going to eat next and worry about whether or not the food is on your diet. It is great for portion control and convenience.

I also like the fact that the program includes an aspect of group support. During the weigh-ins and motivational sessions, you can ask questions of others and learn more about their weight loss and what is working for them. There's accountability there as well; when you know you are going to step on the scale in front of all your colleagues and friends who are also on the diet, you don't want to be the only one who hasn't lost weight. It's like the popular TV show, *The Biggest Loser*. Sometimes the contestants want to give up, but because they don't want to let their team down, they continue to push themselves. That kind of group support is helpful in weight loss, and it is one of the benefits of Jenny Craig.

The downside? It can get expensive because you are paying for the program as well as the prepackaged and prepared foods. It is also not a short program—it's not something you do for a couple of weeks and then finish. A lot of people are on it for a good two years before they see the weight loss they need or want, and they are paying an average of $70 to $100 dollars per week. Now, this is relatively inexpensive if you consider the cost of purchasing food or eating out daily, but low-income dieters can't ordinarily afford it.

The other problem with this program is that because the food is prepackaged and prepared, you do not learn to choose and prepare healthy foods on your own. I worry that when patients finish with the diet, they'll return to former eating and cooking habits because they never learned new ones. So while Jenny Craig is great for convenience, portion control, and consistent weigh loss, it does not do a good job of teaching you how to maintain a lifestyle of healthy eating. For more detailed information on Jenny Craig, go to www.jennycraig.com.

NUTRISYSTEM

Nutrisystem is very similar to Jenny Craig, except that its prepackaged meals are prepared according to the glycemic index. In other words, the diet tries to eliminate bad carbohydrates. Although there are no weekly weigh-ins and no motivational sessions with a weight loss counselor and other dieters, what you do get is the benefit of portion control and convenience. Nutrisystem does offer coaches to talk you through dieting issues and encourage you over the phone, but I believe that the weekly in-person weigh-ins have a stronger impact.

The problems with this diet are similar to Jenny Craig: it's around the same cost, sometimes a little less, but you again run into the issue of not learning to shop for and prepare your own food. Also, management at Nutrisystem admits that only 20 percent of customers actually take advantage of the phone counseling services. Nevertheless, some people have found success with it because it works for their lifestyle. For more information on Nutrisystem, go to www.nutrisystem.com.

THE RICHARD SIMMONS DIET

Richard Simmons designed this diet program based on his own experiences with weight loss. He is well known as a (somewhat eccentric) dance and exercise fanatic, using workout videos to reach others. Now he has expanded his program to be a Web-based experience. When you join his online "Clubhouse," you can pay a monthly or yearly fee and access Richard's Sweatin' videos, get exercise advice, participate in online chats, join the message board community, find recipes, use his restaurant guides to help with food choices when dining out, create shopping lists, maintain an updated progress chart, and keep an online journal.

It can certainly be motivating to see Richard Simmons, who is in his sixties, exercising, dancing, and still releasing new workout videos. His program uses guidelines from the American Diabetes Association and encourages healthy eating according to its recommendations. The monthly or annual membership fees can get expensive, but some may enjoy being a part of something he is affiliated with, since he has had such success with weight loss and maintained it over many years. I have recommended the program for patients with emotional eating issues, since Richard's website deals with emotional and compulsive eaters and people with eating disorders. For more detailed information on the Richard Simmons Diet, go to www.richardsimmons.com.

THE BEST LIFE PLAN

The Best Life Plan was created by Bob Greene, Oprah Winfrey's trainer. I like this diet for one simple reason: it isn't really a diet.

Greene broke this plan into three phases. During the first phase, you are encouraged to cut back on your bad habits; if you eat fried foods, reduce the portion size. If you don't exercise, start exercising! The plan encourages small changes. You're not told that you can't eat a certain type of food; you're just told to cut back. If you eat French fries five times a week, cut it down to one or two. That's Phase 1, which lasts for about a month. Many people don't see a lot of weight loss here, but they are not gaining weight, either.

The second phase of the diet holds the more aggressive lifestyle changes. At this point, Greene tells you that you cannot have any of those bad foods anymore. Stop the chips, stop the fried chicken, and increase the exercise! Greene advises you to focus on this phase for another four weeks, or you can extend it even longer because this is where you start to see weight loss. You can stay in this phase for as long as you need to in order to lose all the weight that you want to lose.

The third and final phase is called the Lifetime Commitment phase, which says that for the rest of your life, you are going to maintain the commitment to your health. You are not going to pick up your bad eating habits again, and you are going to continue to exercise, albeit maybe not with the same intensity that you were showing in Phase 2. For instance, if you were working out five times a week, now you can work out three times a week to maintain the weight loss.

On the Best Life Plan, Greene never really tells you how much to eat or how much not to eat—there is no calorie counting. He just encourages quality control and stresses the necessity of staying active and continuing these habits for a lifetime. The occasional splurge is also allowed; that way, you don't feel as if you can never have fried chicken again!

The good thing about this program is that it gradually transforms your old eating and exercising habits into new, healthy ones. Also, since it's not really a diet, you don't have to spend a lot of money on specialty ingredients for strictly laid out meals.

As far as criticism goes, some people complain that it's a slow process—who wants to go a whole month without seeing weight loss when you're *really* trying to lose weight? But the average patient needs those first few weeks to make small,

The good thing about this program is that it gradually transforms your old eating and exercising habits into new, healthy ones.

healthier lifestyle changes. I tell patients that, okay, they may not lose anything, but they won't gain either. And if you think about it, if you were continuing the way you had been, you probably would have gained another few pounds—so not gaining actually puts you those few pounds ahead! But we don't think about it like that—if you want to see weight loss, you want to see weight loss. We all like quick fixes, and I suspect many dieters get frustrated by the gradual nature of the program and quit before those good habits take hold, which is unfortunate.

My results: As a doctor, I already knew which foods to eat and which not to eat, so I bypassed the first month of the plan, though I did take Greene's advice about increasing my exercise. I would say that patients who do well in the second phase might lose about a pound a week. So it's not an aggressive weight loss method, but it teaches good habits for a lifetime, which is why I recommend it to patients. For more detailed information on the Best Life Plan, go to www.thebestlife.com.

WEIGHT WATCHERS PROGRAM

Weight Watchers can be a complex program if you're unfamiliar with its systems. However, once you join, either through meeting sites or online, everything is explained to you.

At the meeting sites, new members are assigned a coach or group leader, so you're not on your own. The coach or leader is someone who has completely finished the program and maintained his or her goal weight for at least a year, so you also benefit from their knowledge and experience.

When I say Weight Watchers is complex, I mean they expect you to count your carbs, count your "points," maintain food portion control, and attend weekly meetings. There is also online support and handout support materials.

The points system is the most important element of Weight Watchers. Members are assigned a certain number of points a day that they are permitted to eat. This number is determined by your sex, age, activity level, whether you are pregnant or nursing, your height, and current weight. There are points attached to all of these factors, and once you answer all these questions, your Weight Watchers coach or a special calculator called WW Digital Points Calculator adds up the points associated with your responses and determines your allowed points per day.

When I calculated my allowed points on the Weight Watchers program, I was allotted 25 points per day. So what does that 25 points really mean? For example, toast has 1 point, two tablespoons of mayonnaise have 2 points, two lean bacon strips have 3 points, a cup of spaghetti has 7, a cheeseburger 12, and so on. Weight Watchers has allocated the points to every food by using another formula, which is taught to customers so they can always calculate any food they come across by themselves. It is based on the food's total calories, fat grams, and fiber content. The program requires you to track your points and choose foods that will keep you in your point range for the day. However, there are also 35 "fun" points you can use per week if you desire. Points change, too—the more weight you lose, the fewer points you can have in a day, so you must adjust your eating to your current weight and point requirements all the time; otherwise, you might stop losing.

To help avoid plateaus and keep motivated, you should take advantage of the weekly meetings, weigh-ins, and motivational sessions with your weight loss counselor. Every time you hit a milestone, Weight Watchers recognizes your efforts with a milestone gift or award, which makes many participants feel that their efforts are validated.

I have to say this is one of my favorite programs. Though it can be complicated, the fact that you are assigned a coach and do not have to go through the weight loss journey alone is very encouraging. I have seen patients lose a consistent two pounds a week if they are sticking to the program. Yes, you have to learn this method, but the program teaches you many healthy eating habits along the way. When you get used to recognizing what is good for you and what is not, you begin looking at food differently, supporting the larger lifestyle changes I encourage. At around $12 a week, the cost of Weight Watchers is also quite reasonable. The more convenient online version may cost $5 more per week. There is also an initial sign-on fee of around $30. You may occasionally get this fee waived during promotional sessions, such as the beginning of the year. The only caveat is true for most diets: once you reach your goal weight, you must not return to your previous eating habits or stop exercising. Otherwise, the weight loss will not be maintained. For more information on Weight Watchers, go to www.weightwatchers.com.

FAD DIETS

Because they're out there and you've likely considered (if not tried) them, I also want to cover a few fad diets. Fad diets are those that quickly enter our culture and often just as quickly disappear. Many times, they play on our deepest wish: instant gratification. *Lose weight fast! Keep it off for good! Never feel hungry again!*

THE CABBAGE SOUP DIET

This diet is exactly what it sounds like: for seven days, you just eat cabbage soup—all you can eat—morning, noon, and night, with certain fruits and vegetables added on certain days. We don't even know who the author of this diet is because there are so many variations out there. So "they" promise you can lose up to 15 pounds in one week, though most patients average a loss of 10 pounds in a week. Now, "they" also say that you should not continue on this diet longer than those seven days, or you might start having electrolyte problems and other issues from not eating any other nutrients.

A weight loss of 10 pounds a week is not surprising here. Even if you eat this soup non-stop, all day long, it will provide a maximum of 800–1,000 calories. For someone who normally eats 3,000 calories per day, it is a huge reduction, so, of course, weight loss is experienced. The problem is that the first 10 pounds that come off the body that rapidly are usually just water weight. Once you stop the Cabbage Soup Diet and go back to eating regularly—not even overeating—you start to gain the weight back. Of course, you will! You didn't lose fat, nor did you build muscle.

I admit it: I tried this diet. I just wanted to have a "boost," or jump-start of some kind on the scale, so badly … The best part of this diet is that it only lasted seven days! I lost about five pounds, which came right back only two days after resuming normal eating (not excess eating). I didn't like this diet because it didn't emphasize adding exercising to your routine, nor were there any behavior tips or advice for changing your lifestyle. There were also no tips for adjusting your eating habits after that week, which does a disservice to someone who needs a legitimate lifestyle change. However, if you want to get quick pounds off before an event or kick-start a longer diet plan, it is something to try. Warning: people say it makes them super gassy, so if you're brave enough to try it for quick weight loss, you'd better be prepared to stay home for a week!

THE FAT FLUSH DIET

This is basically a detox program plus weight loss plan that is divided into three phases. The first phase, which lasts 1–2 weeks, limits your calorie intake to 1,200 calories per day. During the second phase, you can increase your calories to 1,500, and then you can stay at this level for as long as you need to lose all the weight that you need to lose. Finally, you move to the maintenance phase, during which you can start eating over 1,500 calories.

Now, the diet does restrict your foods, and you must eat from its list of allowed foods to make up those particular calories. While it is a rather balanced diet in terms of its proteins, carbs, and other food groups, it is very particular. This diet also emphasizes daily exercise, which is good, but it requires you to have a minimum of eight hours of scheduled sleep a day to see maximum effectiveness. The diet also includes a "detox" aspect, which includes flax oil, special cranberry juice, and other supplements that are supposed to detoxify your system. Also, you must buy these supplements directly from the website, and they finish rather quickly so you have to keep buying more.

I would not recommend this diet to my patients. First of all, I don't believe in the detoxifying process. Our intestinal tract is naturally designed to detoxify by itself as long as we eat plenty of fiber and drink enough water daily. Secondly, it can get pretty expensive. The diet is so detailed that you must have the book that sells for about $25, plus the detoxifying system that costs about $75, plus the protein powder, which costs another $45, plus other vitamins and supplements. This diet is also very restrictive. Expecting any patient who comes in eating 3,000 calories a day to cut down to only 1,200 calories a day on their own is absurd. For those who can restrict themselves and stay on that low number of calories for the required time, it may be doable. And if the diet didn't have the "detoxifying" portion, I might say this is not so bad. But due to the nature of the plan, I believe that part of the weight loss may come from the patient becoming dehydrated and in semi-starvation mode. I have never, nor will I ever, try this diet. For more information, visit www.annlouise.com.

LIQUID DIETS

I come across liquid diets often, as they are recommended for bariatric patients who are preparing for weight loss surgery. I discuss patients' needs and goals with their bariatric surgeons in order to design a diet that would be effective prior to their surgery. Patients are usually required to go on a liquid diet for about two weeks prior to surgery because it helps rapidly lose the fat that has enlarged the liver, shrinking it down for a safer surgery. These patients often see rapid weight and fat loss during these diets, up to 15 pounds in two weeks (but most of it is from water weight).

Other liquid diets, like Slim-Fast and Optifast, have had some staying power and popularity. (Oprah lost around 67 pounds on Optifast in about four months). These drinks are meant to be meal replacements. Some people who do well with prepackaged foods do well with Slim-Fast and Optifast because they are ready to go. Every time you are hungry, just pop a top and drink. You don't eat any real food during these diets, and you limit yourself to less than 1,200 calories a day.

Like Oprah, many lose a significant amount of weight in a relatively short time, but does it last? Oprah looked great, felt great, and she was working out during that time in 1988—and then she reached her goal, started eating "real food" again, stopped exercising as hard, and eventually regained all the weight and then some. Oprah is always in the public eye and has plenty of money to hire a permanent personal trainer—yet she regained the weight. What does that tell you about these diets? In fact, I have yet to see someone who has kept their weight off after finishing a liquid diet and resuming normal eating habits.

That's because there are not guidelines for maintaining the weight loss outside of returning to the diet once you gain it back. It can be used as a jumpstart to another slower paced diet, though. For more information, go to www.slim-fast.com or www.optifast.com.

P90X

I'll use this as an example of a program combining diet and exercise, but there are many such programs out there.

You've probably seen the infomercials. If so, you know that people have actually been very successful with this weight loss method. P90X requires you to exercise for one hour every day for 90 days. The program includes an exercise DVD that shows you exactly what exercises to do each day. It also tells you which foods to eat, laying out all three meals and snacks in between. The goal of the program is to transform people in those 90 days: their bodies from the exercise and their minds from the recommended lifestyle. The program is great and it is effective. And it is tough. Really tough.

I tried P90X. I lasted about two and a half weeks and then could not do anymore. I mean, *physically,* I just could not continue. The exercises are not easy. In fact, they are some of the hardest I have ever done, even harder than when my personal trainer was pushing me every day. They require pushups, pull-ups, crunches, and tri-core work; for the patient with limited mobility, this program is very intimidating. Many overweight individuals will not be able to do the program completely right away. Part of the program insert even said this program was for conditioned athletes.

One of the things I did wrong was that I did not start slow and then build up. I went full-on 100 percent on the first day and put all I could into it the first week. By the second week, I skipped a day here and there, and by the third week, I dreaded the workout. I could feel my muscles developing, but for someone starting out, this exercise program would be too rough. There was no start-here, beginners, intermediate, and advanced level; it was just one DVD for each muscle group: abs, back, chest, yoga, etc. The diet itself was great, however. It encouraged healthy choices in food and took the question out of what you were going to eat because it was very clear about what you could and should eat. For more info, go to www.beachbody.com.

Though the diets and weight loss programs covered in this chapter are some of the more popular and often successful ones out there, they are by no means the only ones. I encourage you to do your own research to determine which programs suit your lifestyle the best. And if you doubt that you can make *any* diet fit into your lifestyle, the next chapter will offer some tips!

CHAPTER 8

YOU *CAN* CONTROL YOUR CIRCUMSTANCES

WHEN you've been struggling for years with your weight, it's easy to feel powerless. Powerless to your body, powerless to the world around you, powerless to make a change that will work and that you can keep. But sinking into this kind of passive, helpless mode is what will keep you in this hole. You have more control than you think.

CULTURE

Culture can be a tricky subject to approach when it concerns weight gain: depending on your culture and your own personality, you may find it either very easy or very hard to reconcile your culture and your health. Part of this is because, as I've mentioned, "health" may be defined differently from one culture to the next, and you may find yourself at odds with what your culture and family believe is the best way to live. In fact, your attempt to resolve your health and weight issues may actually cause you to feel alienated from the rest of your family.

For example, if you come from a family that fries most foods, and then you invite them over for Thanksgiving and choose to bake your turkey rather than fry it, they may wonder what is wrong with you! Or if you choose not to partake in some of the foods at a typical family gathering, it's possible for people to feel insulted or even judged by your attempt to eat healthfully. The best thing to do in situations like this is to educate your family and explain that the doctor has said you are cutting at least 10 years from your life by continuing to eat this way. Being up front with your family about the changes you have decided to make may be difficult, but it can be crucial to your success.

HOW MY CULTURE INFLUENCED MY DIET

My Nigerian diet growing up was very different from the American diet. I was raised by my paternal uncle and his wife in what was considered an average income family in Nigeria at that time. The food was always home-cooked, and we did not have as many choices; whatever was on the dinner table was what we ate. The meals normally consisted of a large portion of carbohydrates and very little protein—half or even a quarter of what is recommended in the U.S. Trust me, it's not because we didn't *want* more protein; access was limited, so it boiled down to cost. The carbs were more filling and a lot cheaper.

We ate three square meals a day, with no snacking in between. No indulging in a bag of chips and soda just because they were around and you were bored while watching television. There were not that many fresh vegetables in our diet (again due to high cost), but fruits were everywhere, ripening and falling from trees—free for us to pick as we went along. I remember in my middle school days, if you were hungry, you would just pick whatever was growing on the trees around you. And if you were walking along the streets and there were mangos or guava dropping, you could take them and eat for free. A huge difference from the vending machines in U.S. schools!

At age 16, I relocated to be with my parents and siblings in the U.S. It actually took me quite a while to adjust to eating American food. I didn't like a lot of things initially; cheese and milk products for example, were not part of our daily diet in Nigeria. I remember seeing cheese on everything in America and thinking, *I can't eat that stuff!* But after about two years of living here, I began to acquire the taste for American food. Breyers vanilla ice cream with real bean specks was my first love. Of course, my siblings, who had lived here their whole lives, preferred American food—the French fries, the chips, and soda—over the Nigerian meals my mom made, because that was what they ate in school. My youngest brother, in fact, did not at all want the African foods. So at times, my siblings would eat separately from the rest of the family because they had acquired a taste for fattier junk foods and sugary drinks.

My mom's career choice did not help matters: she cooks and caters professionally for intercontinental events, and food was always abundant in our house. Her menus consisted of African, American, Italian, Greek, and Asian foods. She cooked so well and so much that there were always delicious samples left over to try. Many major holidays were held at our house because my relatives could always count on some good food being there. Preparations for these events would start days before, and she cooked for hours upon hours, peeling potatoes, chopping up ingredients, and getting ready for the feast. To satisfy everyone, she made both American and Nigerian foods, and many of them would be high in calories and cooked with lots of oils and fats. One snack I remember her making was called a Puff Puff, which was basically fried flour and sugar. They were called Puff Puffs because people believed that eating a lot of them would make you puffy or fat. (True enough!) Of course, we had to try everything my mother cooked, and we ate and ate until we felt like we were going to fall over. Then came naptime. When we woke, we ate again! It was a terrible (but delicious) cycle.

ADAPTING MY CULTURE

As with many Americans, weight is an issue for my family. Many of us have had to adjust our eating habits and diets to compensate for the weight gain. Just like I have, my siblings also have struggled with it, and so has my mom. It actually became easier for me to manage my own weight when I was no longer living at home. I had full control over what I was eating, what was cooked, and how I was cooking it. Family visits, however, were another story.

Obviously, a part of my family culture is that when we get together, we eat! During one visit, when I first explained that I was on a diet, they were shocked at the restrictions—no sugar, no carbs, no oil, no fat. Only lean protein, fresh fruits, and vegetables. And when they came to visit and I served them salads and salmon, they exclaimed, "Where's the real food?" They'd raid my fridge only to find it stocked with fresh fruits and veggies. Then they knew I was serious.

Once I changed my eating habits, I needed to explain that I could not continue to eat the way that was causing me to gain weight. "I've made changes to try to live a better and healthier lifestyle," I told them. "I've had to cut certain things out of my diet. This is what I eat now, and this is what I have to offer you." I had to be firm with educating them, or I would end up cooking their way every time they came around, and that simply would not work for me. Now I use it as an opportunity to show my family that food cooked differently can taste just as good and be healthier for them.

Plus, once they saw my weight loss results, my family realized that what I was doing was working and didn't want to be the ones to mess it up for me. My mother was especially supportive and asked me what I was allowed to eat on my diet so that when visiting them, she would make sure there were things I could eat in the house. Once my mom was on board, everyone else was, too, and that kind of support makes it easier to stick to my diet when I visit. My sister and I even went on a little competition to see who would lose the most weight sticking to the diet and exercising.

So my advice? Let your family know you've changed your diet, not just to lose weight but to get healthier. For family in your home, explain that the changes you are making are going to be permanent, not just for the diet. Tell them that this is the way you're all going to be living from now on—be firm, and try to get everyone on board. Be up front and offer up healthier suggestions and activities.

Do you have a family reunion coming up? Do you typically barbeque and everyone indulges in the unhealthy foods? Why not change it up a bit? Plan a sporting event or some outside games at the park and have gift cards and monetary rewards for the winners. The reunion should be about sharing time together as a family. It does not have to revolve around eating unhealthy foods! And this way, you don't have to worry about jeopardizing all your efforts for one event.

THE ENVIRONMENT

You can't always change the environment to work better for you and your eating habits, but you can certainly make changes in your own life to adapt, rather than conform, to your surroundings.

REMOVE YOURSELF FROM TEMPTATION

For me, it probably helped a great deal that I was not living at home when I began my weight loss journey. I was able to control my environment and limit temptations. In fact, I *claimed* my own environment. First, I made sure I didn't have any junk food around. I cleaned out the pantry and refrigerator, replacing junk food with healthy options. That way, even when I felt like cheating, all I had in my refrigerator were apples, blueberries, crunchy sugar snap peas, and baby carrots. As for work, I did not carry cash with me, so there was no way I was going to run out and buy anything from a vending machine. And I knew I would never borrow money from a colleague to buy it, either. Clean and change your environment to work best for you.

SMALL STEPS CAN STILL MAKE YOU SWEAT

You don't have to run a marathon to introduce exercise to your environment! If you live or work in a place with an elevator, start taking the stairs if you are not going up more than three flights. Leave the car at home when you're only going a few blocks. This adds a few extra steps to your daily count. If you like playing video games, incorporate ones like Wii Sports to your routine. You'd be surprised how much exercise you can get from the Wii—we've actually made it a family event and have worked up a sweat after playing some of the games!

EDUCATE YOURSELF

Obesity is more prevalent in lower-income groups than in higher-income groups. If you can further your education—either by going back to college or grad school, earning a certificate, or attending seminars and voluntary courses at work—you could increase your income. At that point, chances are some other things will change in your environment that lead to healthier options becoming available. But in the meantime ...

CREATE YOUR OWN HEALTHY OPTIONS

If your environment is lacking some of the healthier amenities you wish you had, create healthy programs that will work for you! My colleague told me that a small group of people in her neighborhood came together and decided to start growing fruits or vegetables in their backyards. They made their chosen food as organic and healthy as possible, and then exchanged it amongst each other just the way a local farmers market might do. You might grow tomatoes, the Johnsons down the road might have a lemon tree, and the Ramirez family has an herb garden. Exchanging excess fruits and veggies can save a lot of money on groceries, and you're eating healthier! Plus, growing your own food is an opportunity to learn healthier, tastier ways of cooking fresh meals. A win-win situation for everyone! Just Google "neighborhood produce exchange" for detailed ideas on how to start one in your neighborhood.

> **Growing your own food is an opportunity to learn healthier, tastier ways of cooking meals.**

COMBATING THE FOOD INDUSTRY

Can we blame our obesity entirely on the food industry? No, but we have to be wary consumers, armed with the knowledge that the food industry knows how to bring us back for more. Through clever marketing and, of course, hitting our reward centers, the industry makes money off our consumption of its products. We have to remember that they want into our pockets, again and again. A burger is not just a burger. I'm not suggesting that we stop eating out altogether, but I would try to pick restaurants that are more health conscious.

Also, realize that *it is okay for you to customize your food*, even at a restaurant. You *can* say you want your chicken grilled without the heavy sauce. You're paying for your food, so you should be able to pick what you want and adjust it according to your dietary needs. For instance, I had lunch the other day at a chain restaurant. As I looked over the menu options, I realized that I didn't want my salad prepared the way it was described. Yes, it was just a salad, but the ingredients included a "crusted" chicken (synonym for battered and fried), with confectioners' sugar on top. I asked the waiter to grill my chicken instead and put it in my salad with the dressing on the side. I asked for the vegetables, which I knew would be steamed in butter, to be steamed without any sauces or oils. My waiter and chef might not like me, but my order was prepared exactly the way I wanted it, and I ate lunch without feeling guilty afterward. Sometimes you just have to spell out what you want!

THE SUPER-SIZED PROBLEM

American portions are *big*. They're two, sometimes even three, sizes more than we need, and there's a point when you have to take control over how much food is on your plate. At first, if you can't resist or cut down large portions at restaurants, you may have to plan ahead and bring your own food to work. But eventually, you need to learn to say no when you're offered the super-sized version of a meal, whether it's at a fast food joint or a sit-down restaurant. For the latter, that might mean splitting a meal with the person you're eating dinner with, or packing half of it away at the *beginning of your meal* and saving it for the next day.

In order to win this war, you *have* to be proactive. You must be the educated consumer and make healthier choices. It's okay if you want to splurge every now and then—everyone does that—but remember: eating out does not excuse you from the same rules you try to live by at home. You may not be able to control everything, but you're the master of your own behavior.

BLAME IT ON THE GENES

Genetics is the most difficult "circumstance" to address because some aspects of the way your own body functions really are out of your control. It's your genes versus your behavior here, and the first side has home team advantage. However, just as in sports, smart, intentional plays are the key to success.

First, you need to stay active. And not just as active as an average person—you need to stay even *more* active than the average person. If it has been determined that your genes make you more likely to gain weight than someone else, you must do more than the average recommended activity level of 150 minutes per week. I also tell my patients that they need to calculate their BMR, or basal metabolic rate, because we really need to know what their specific daily caloric requirement is. (Refer to Chapter 2 for the Harris-Benedict equation.)

For example, let's say one of my patients needs 2,700 calories to maintain his weight. Unless we know that number, we cannot create an accurate and effective diet plan to help him lose weight. But once I know that number, I can say, "Okay, you can afford to cut down on 350 calories every day." Since 3,500 calories is equal to one pound, cutting 350 calories a day adds up, and by staying active, my patient will start losing weight at a rate of one to two pounds per week. If I had assumed that this patient needed the same 2,000 calories as a similarly built man, I would have cut his calories too dramatically or not enough and set him up for failure.

Of course, as well as staying active, I also recommend a healthy diet. You have to eat right, eat the right amount, and eat at the right time. And it is even more important for you, because you are obesogenic!

GET SUPPORT
I feel it's even more important for someone struggling with genetic weight gain to find a support group of people with similar issues rather than feeling helpless and accepting their "fate." It helps to interact with others who understand your situation and can be there for you, without judging you in a way that others might. You can search for online support groups in your area. Weight loss blogs and websites are also great resources to help you deal with your weight problems and goals. Some of the ones I've used are www.3fatchicks.com, www.hcgdietinfo.com, and www.dailystrength.org. Find a support group whose

objectives match with your own personal reasons for seeking support and encouragement.

Personally, I found many of these online weight loss communities and blogs to be a cheerleader for me. Like a supportive family, we worked toward the same goal together: losing the weight that had been plaguing us for so long. I signed up for the groups even before I started my diet. I learned so much from reading and hearing about other people's experiences with their own diets. Many questions I had were already answered by other users at some point, and I could find those answers by just reading some of the archived discussions.

DEALING WITH METABOLISM

If your metabolism really is causing your weight gain or preventing you from losing weight, the goal is to help your metabolism work more efficiently—that is, burn more calories and decrease your metabolic age. The first step is to make sure your doctor does blood work to check for medical conditions that can slow down your efforts, such as thyroid issues and Cushing's syndrome, a disease caused by the body having too much cortisol. This helps ensure your metabolism is not being affected by these treatable disorders.

Now, we can't turn back the clock and do anything about your chronological age, but you *can* help your metabolic age by exercising. You can lose all the weight you want, but if you don't exercise, your metabolic age doesn't change. This is because exercise builds healthier muscles, which in turn burn more calories and improve your metabolic age rating. (Metabolic age is a relatively new term used to describe one's overall fitness, and is calculated by comparing your BMR to the average BMR of others in your chronological age group.)

Some women are scared of building muscles through exercise—they tell me all the time that they do not want to "bulk up." Instead, I encourage them to do the type of exercise that gives you lean muscle, as an alternative to the types that give you bulky muscle. To get bulky muscle, the way men might, you lift really heavy weights and do few repetitions; to get lean muscle, you lift light weights and do lots of repetitions. I usually encourage women who are afraid of bulking up to lift no more than 10–15-pound weights. Start with 8 repetitions per set and then work your way up to 15, with a goal of three sets. This will make your muscles lean and slim but still burn calories and increase metabolism.

Sleep is also crucial for keeping your metabolism running properly and maintaining weight. Your body is able to get rid of toxins and repair itself during sleep. Just like a tired person is slower and less efficient, so is a tired cell that has not had the chance to rest enough. The delicate balance of hormone secretion (such as cortisol, leptin, and ghrelin) and glucose handling can be disrupted when the body is sleep deprived, leading to increased stress, increased appetite, and weight gain. I experienced this firsthand during my residency days of 30-plus hours straight of working without any sleep. I was most stressed and hungry after my shifts and definitely gained the most weight around this time. Go to bed early if you can; not only will you have a great morning after getting eight hours of sleep, but your metabolism will also thank you by functioning more efficiently.

Drinking plenty of water (remember, your urine should be almost clear) during the day is also key, since your cells need water to function. And the more fruits and vegetables you can get in your diet, the better, though most of us also need to supplement with daily multivitamins.

Also, frequent eating can help to keep your metabolism up. (There's something to the 3-Hour Diet, after all.) Eating every few hours makes your body believe it will not need to store everything it takes in because it will be getting more fuel shortly. The body is tricked, for lack of a better word, into burning more calories. The reason we think there might be truth to this is that this is how people ate before the industrial age. They never sat down to eat three big meals a day, and obesity was far less an issue then.

As a related aside, the skinniest girl I've ever met eats every two hours! I asked her how she could stay so thin when she was eating all the time, and she said she did not eat *meals*, per se; instead, she nibbled throughout the day. She might drink a V8 tomato drink, followed by a quarter of a bagel two hours later, then some carrots two hours after that, and so on. Granted, she was not consuming a crazy amount of calories, but eating frequently worked for her. If your metabolism is the issue, it could work for you, too.

YOUR TURN

What I've offered in this chapter are suggestions that are fully within your reach. So, reach! And if it turns out you need something more dramatic, Chapter 9 will cover some alternative solutions that just might be right for you.

ALTERNATIVE WEIGHT LOSS SOLUTIONS AND "SOLUTIONS"

WHEN you've been trying for months or years to lose a significant amount of weight, it can be tempting to turn to alternative solutions. Many of these are actually beneficial, and some are necessary—but others play on your desperation and market a solution that is ineffective at best and dangerous at worst. It's important to know the difference.

THE TOXIN TALK

Some people (various chiropractors, naturopaths, nutritionists, and assorted food faddists) believe you gain weight because there are up to 25 pounds of excess waste and toxins lingering in your colon. They state that undigested meats and other foods we eat form hardened feces and accumulate for months (or even years) on the walls of the large intestine, blocking it from absorbing or eliminating properly. This, according to them, builds a layer of so-called "mucoid plaque" in the colon, causing clogging, constipation, and a breeding ground for bacterial growth. These proponents portray the large intestine as a sewage system that becomes a septic tank if neglected. Some even state that there are worms and parasites there, growing and attacking the immune system and leading to many diseases.

This is their reasoning behind colonic cleansing, especially during weight loss efforts—the idea that if you can flush your body of toxins and the buildup, you will lose weight. Some even think that while you're losing weight, all the fat you are releasing gets dumped into the colon along with the toxins and needs something to stick lest it just get reabsorbed into the body, defeating the whole purpose. Frankly, this is ludicrous. What many of these people don't realize is that the body is truly fascinating in its functions. It has the ability to *detox* itself of toxins and other matter that doesn't belong. The organs that are employed for the elimination of toxins are the kidneys, liver, colon, skin, and lungs. Toxins from the body are eliminated through urine, feces, perspiration, and exhalation. Part of the job of the liver is to break down harmful toxins into harmless byproducts that can easily be eliminated from the body in the form of stools or urine.

The body has the ability to detox itself of toxins and other matter that doesn't belong, using the kidneys, liver, colon, skin, and lungs.

The colon is a hollow 40-inch-long tube whose principal functions are to transport food from the small intestine to the large intestine, and then transport food wastes from there to the rectum for final elimination. It also absorbs minerals and water along the way. Hundreds of beneficial bacteria like Lactobacillus acidophilus live naturally in the colon to help reduce toxin activity, boost the immune system, and reduce side effects of undigestible foods. There is no medical evidence that detox diets or colonic cleansing actually remove any toxin from the body. Direct observation of the colon during surgical procedures such as colonoscopies or autopsies show no evidence that any hardened feces accumulate on the intestinal walls.

Those who buy into the colonic toxin theory claim that by "cleansing" your colon, you will improve your health by washing out all that gunk and bacteria from your body. They also say you will lose anywhere from 5–10 pounds after just one treatment, enhance your immune system, gain energy, and reduce bloating. Some even claim it cures cancer and numerous other conditions. A miracle!

Well, as I already explained, the colon is designed to naturally eliminate its own waste. Increasing the number of bowel movements every day doesn't affect the weight; your small intestine has already absorbed all the nutrients from the food before it reaches the large intestine. The only stuff left is the material your body says it doesn't need. Most of the time, that's roughages your body simply can't process.

And that so-called "unnatural mucoid layer" in the colon? Its job is to keep unwanted processes from re-entering into the bloodstream. It is actually mucus secreted by individual cells or glands lining the inside of the colon to aid in digestion and protection. That means the body puts it there naturally—it is not waste from food; it is there to *prevent* waste and substance from re-entering your body. Cleaning it out with forceful laxatives could really hurt you.

The other reason I disagree with this theory is that the intestinal lining is designed to shed daily, and the typical life cycle of these cells is about three to seven days, so there is no buildup to be cleaned.

When you use colon cleansing products, it's the contents of the product itself that are actually being eliminated from your body. That is, the product you just consumed produces the very condition that it claims to treat. Some people have reported expelling large amounts of what they claim to be feces that have accumulated on the intestinal wall. However, experts believe these are simply "casts" formed by the fiber contained in the "cleansing" products. Many of these products contain psyllium and bentonite clays, which are bulk-forming laxatives that simply absorb water in the colon and form a rope-like mess that then comes out of your gut with some small amount of stool on its outside. You see it and think you've just gotten rid of all your toxins and weight woes—genius, if you ask me!—but in fact, your body is simply expelling what you put in it.

Yes, after using these products, you will lose weight—but it's water weight, not fat. The product just absorbs a tremendous amount of water from your body. The problem is that most people who use these cleansers are looking for instant gratification—to lose a few pounds before a big event. But if an *obese* person uses the product and loses five pounds, he thinks that if he keeps using the product, he will keep losing five pounds every time. When this doesn't happen, he ends up frustrated. Patients like this come into my office dehydrated, with cramps and electrolyte abnormalities, and some may even have bowel perforation, which can be deadly.

As a final argument, many of the ingredients in colon cleansers are not regulated by the FDA because they claim to be natural compounds and herbs; the manufacturers can put anything in them that they think might work as long as its "natural." How is this even possible? Natural herbs don't hurt, right? Well, ask the families of people who have died from colonic cleansing complications. If that's not terrifying, I don't know what is.

Want to hear a secret? You can achieve the same thing as colonic cleansers by increasing the amount of fiber, fruits, and vegetables in your diet and avoiding processed foods! Your body can't break down fiber, so it travels through your colon and aids in removing waste. This is a healthier, cheaper way to "cleanse your colon." In fact, the only appropriate use for colon cleansing is for a colonoscopy, which is where the colon is completely cleaned and examined for signs of cancer.

PRESCRIPTION WEIGHT LOSS

During my weight loss journey, I decided to look into prescription weight loss. Specifically, I looked at Alli, which is available over the counter. Other medications available for weight loss need a doctor's prescription and work as stimulants, making your heart work faster. Alli works by stopping your body from absorbing the fat in the food you eat. However, there are a lot of gastrointestinal side effects, such as abdominal cramping, bloating, gas, leakage, oily stools, and diarrhea, because Alli stops the release of digestive juices that help break down fat. Plus, when I looked at the average amount of weight lost, it was a measly five percent when combined with diet and exercise for over a year. For me, that would have been about 12 pounds after a year of being on the medication. I had at least 40 pounds to lose, and at that rate, it would take up to four years. That was not going to work, especially if the weight came back once I stopped taking the medication. Also, Alli's long-term safety profile has not been established past a few short years.

As for other FDA approved prescription drugs, I was scared to put any of them into my body. You've heard of them—Fen Phen, Ephedra, Meridia. What happens with many of these drugs is that the FDA approves them and then, a few years later, pulls them off the market because they are causing health problems such as heart attacks, severe hypertension, heart failure, stroke, irregular heart-beats, seizure, insomnia, strokes, and even death. I was not going to put my body at risk or give myself another problem while trying to lose weight.

That, in a nutshell, is my problem with a lot of FDA approved weight loss drugs. If I put a patient on a diet and weight loss medication but she develops hypertension, heart disease, or congestive heart failure from the medicine, it's not worth it. As I've said, a diet or a weight loss method should *improve* your health, not impair it. You shouldn't have to worry that your diet will give you another medical problem or issue down the line. I do not believe that any of the current FDA approved drugs are the answer to weight loss. Even when they help patients lose some weight, the patients usually gain the weight right back after ceasing the medication.

Phentermine is an amphetamine appetite suppressant prescribed a lot lately by doctors for weight loss in over-weight and obese patients. It is used for a limited time (FDA recommends only three months) to speed weight loss in people who are exercising and eating a low-calorie diet. Phentermine can be habit forming, causing you to need higher doses as time goes on to get the same effect.

Other people might simply stop responding to it. If it is not combined with diet and exercise, you won't see weight loss and you get the side effects, which can include dry mouth, unpleasant taste, constipation, increased blood pressure, heart palpitations, restlessness, tremor or nervousness, insomnia, and/or chest pain. It is not recommended for patients with heart disease and moderate to severe hypertension, which a lot of overweight and obese patients suffer from.

In general, I don't think prescription weight loss is the answer.

LIPOSUCTION

While it is technically true that you can "lose weight" through liposuction, I don't consider it a *weight loss* method; it is more of a cosmetic surgery. Surgeons use liposuction to literally suck out pounds of fat in a localized area. They focus on one small area at a time in order to make sure it looks as even and symmetrical as possible. Some surgeons are braver than others, and if you have a lot of subcutaneous fat to lose, they might remove anywhere from 5 to 40 percent. For severely obese patients, up to 10 pounds can be removed in one procedure session. Additional sessions are usually necessary for other specific areas you wish to target for fat removal.

Liposuction is a procedure that requires super specialized surgeons—plastic surgeons—who have gone through five years of general surgery training and an additional two to three years of plastic surgery residency training. This kind of expertise doesn't come cheap!

I don't recommend liposuction to my patients as a weight loss method because it doesn't address any of the underlying behavioral issues nor does it stop the remaining fat cells from secreting substances to recruit more fat cells. *But* it can be useful in patients who have used other weight loss methods to lose the weight but are having trouble with a particular small problem area that just won't go away no matter what (for example, that pad between the knees, love handles, the C-section bulge, etc.).

STOMACH BALLOON

This is one of those weight loss methods whose name fairly accurately represents its function: the stomach balloon works to take up room in your stomach so there is less room for food and you feel full faster. There are two methods to creating this effect—a surgical and a non-surgical option.

In the surgical option, an actual balloon made out of durable elastic (high-quality silicone) is inserted into the stomach. The doctor will insert a camera through the back of your throat and go into your stomach, similar to what he would do if he were checking for stomach ulcers or other conditions like cancer. At the end of the camera is a mechanism to deploy the balloon into your stomach and then fill it with approximately 400–700 milliliters of saline solution or air. The balloon has a self-sealing valve and floats freely inside the stomach, simply taking up space. Once filled, the balloon is too large to pass into the bowel. Common side effects are varying degrees of nausea, vomiting, and abdominal pain. Occasional gastritis (stomach lining irritation) is reported.

The procedure usually takes about 30 minutes to perform. No overnight hospital stay is required. In fact, you can usually go home three hours after the balloon is inserted and inflated. Some doctors prefer a patient stay overnight in the hospital. However, unlike bariatric surgeries, such as lap band, after which certain high-fat foods must be avoided, you can eat all types of foods after gastric ballooning—just in smaller portions. The balloon can be left in place no longer than about six months because erosion by stomach acid can occur. Once removed, the stomach—and many times the patient's appetite—returns to normal.

Weight loss with this method can be up to 35 percent of your excess body weight in six months. By contrast, people tend to lose 50–65 percent with gastric by-pass surgery. **Weight loss can be up to 35% of excess body weight within six months.** This surgical balloon version is not currently approved in the U.S., but it is in parts of Europe, Canada, Australia, Mexico, and South America. It costs about $4,500 U.S. dollars—a fraction of the cost of gastric bypass. But there are some concerns (of course). Besides not being approved in the U.S., the balloon's safety and effectiveness is also not well known. The balloon technique also doesn't significantly reduce ghrelin (the stomach hunger hormone), which gastric bypass surgery suppresses pretty well. There is associated risk of rupture, breakdown from stomach acid, and slippage into the intestines, where it can cause life-threatening obstructions. Long-lasting weight loss may not be enough to make this investment worthwhile. It may have a role, however, for the right patients—such as high-risk obese patients who need to lose weight in order make the actual gastric bypass surgery procedure safer.

The non-surgical method consists of taking a daily formula that, once swallowed, reaches the stomach and absorbs water, thus taking up space and reducing the amount of food it needs to feel full. It gives a gastric bypass effect by leaving only 20 percent of the stomach space for food. It technically lasts for about 10–16 hours a day but may need a boost once or twice throughout the day in some folks. Makers claim you can lose 10–15 pounds a month because you eat less, and the cost is about $500 for a four-month supply if you buy during special promotional seasons. One company that makes this type of formula in the U.S. is Roca Labs. This version claims to be made of "all natural ingredients," so no FDA approval is required. One common side effect is dehydration, as the formula absorbs a large portion of water from the body. So, if you are not constantly drinking fluids to keep up, you might see this happen.

I have never recommended either of these methods for weight loss because there isn't enough data evaluating their effectiveness in the short or long term. The last thing you need is another temporary "solution." A lot of us eat for reasons that have nothing to do with being physically hungry or full, and there will be no effect if you continuously nibble on bad foods thorough out the day.

BARIATRIC SURGERY

Now, I am not a bariatric surgeon, but I believe bariatric surgery is a very effective method of weight loss, and I recommend it to patients who have an extreme amount of weight to lose. Before you decide to follow this road, though, you need to be aware of the potential risks and complications, as well as the medical requirements needed to clear you for surgery.

Patients who would qualify for bariatric surgery have a BMI of at least 40, meaning they have at least 100 pounds of excess body weight to lose. Since a higher BMI is associated with risk factors such as hypertension, diabetes, high cholesterol, liver problems, and obstructive sleep apnea, and weight loss surgery can help reduce all these risks, many insurance companies are now willing to pony up.

Patients who would qualify for bariatric surgery have a BMI of at least 40, meaning they have at least 100 pounds of excess body weight to lose.

Bariatric surgery can also be performed in someone with a BMI of 30 or more as long as they have a second condition that would benefit from the procedure. For instance, if you have a BMI of 30, and you are diabetic and have obstructive sleep apnea, you could potentially qualify for the surgery. However, you could rarely walk into the doctor's office with a BMI of 30 and no other problems and qualify with your insurance company. They simply will not pay for it, since it can run anywhere from $10,000 to $30,000. And since one out of three Americans is obese, insurance companies have to have some qualifications before they will approve the procedure.

If a patient qualifies and decides to move forward with surgery, the surgeon will analyze the patient's anatomy, risk factors, and liver size. Depending on these factors, the surgeon might recommend one of the following three common procedures.

OPTION 1: ROUX-EN-Y GASTRIC BYPASS
This procedure has been around the longest (over 20 years). With it, the stomach is divided into two pouches: a really

small top pouch and a bigger bottom called the body; surgeons divide the stomach by either sewing or stapling. The procedure reduces your stomach to hold about one ounce of food or fluid. Eventually, the stomach will stretch to be able to hold four to six ounces.

This procedure will also divide your small intestine; the surgeon will join the lower piece of the small intestine to the new small top stomach pouch that has just been created. Then the remaining body of the stomach is connected to the remaining part of the small intestine. By doing this, you bypass the part of the small intestine that actually absorbs a lot of the food and its nutrients.

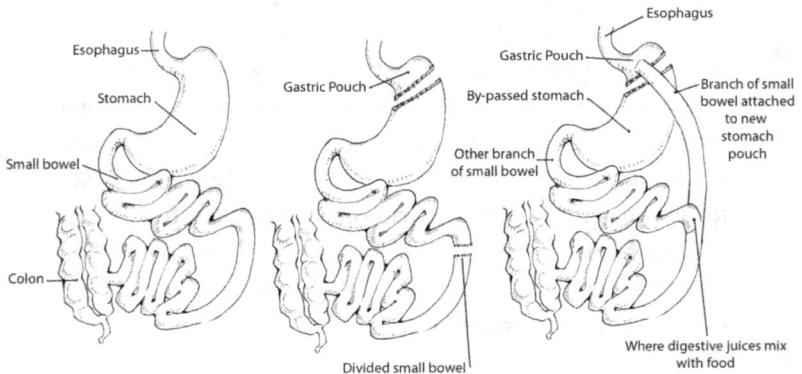

What is accomplished by the procedure is that you get full quickly from very small amounts of food. You also don't absorb a lot of the calories, fat, or nutrients from what you are eating—they basically run right through.

This method is highly durable, and patients maintain their weight loss for many years afterwards. The weight loss is rapid: patients can lose up to 60–80 percent of their excess body weight in the first year. So if a patient weighed 400 pounds with 200 pounds of excess body weight, he will typically lose around 120–160 pounds during that first year. That is a significant amount of weight loss, and the fact that it is maintainable for years makes this a great method.

There are some drawbacks to the procedure, however. This kind of surgery actually bypasses the part of the gas-trointestinal (GI) tract that absorbs a lot of nutrients such as sugars and fats. Patients can therefore develop what we call "dumping syndrome." In this condition, when the patient eats foods such as simple sugars, processed carbs, or raw fats, their body simply can't absorb or use it, so it just dumps it straight into the large intestine, causing ex-plosive diarrhea, nausea, vomiting, stomach cramps, and pain. You may also feel sweaty, dizzy, and shaky. Some people get nauseous and weak, and they have palpita-tions (heart rate goes up). Patients who suffer from this syndrome always know where the closest bathrooms are whenever they go out, and it is an uncomfortable way to live the first year after the surgery. Not everyone will experience the same severity of symptoms, but until you train yourself not to eat certain foods, you have to be cautious.

The bright side of the dumping syndrome is that it forces the patient to start eating healthier since they can't tolerate the unhealthy foods. But because they have bypassed the part of the bowel that absorbs nutrients, they often become deficient in protein and vitamins and have to take lifetime supplements of protein, iron, vitamin B12, and all the things that should have been absorbed from diet by the small intestine. They have to be on daily multivitamins;

at first, some require a double dose to make sure they get everything they need. Sometimes, they are given vitamin B12 shots to bypass the GI tract altogether.

It is also important for women who wish to have children to decide if they want to do this procedure before or after they get pregnant. Preparing your body to have a baby can be difficult when you cannot eat certain things or keep food down. Pregnant women are often nauseated anyway, and this procedure can add another degree of nausea on top of it. We always counsel patients about this, but data does show that women *can* get pregnant after this procedure. In fact, we have found out that, for some, fertility actually increases once excess weight is lost. But it is important to recognize that a person who has undergone this procedure may have a tougher time due to GI issues.

The Roux-en-Y gastric bypass is a very complex and permanent procedure—once the surgeon sews your small intestine to your new smaller stomach, it's done. No going back. Nowadays, the surgical risk associated with this method is less than 0.002 percent, but you must find a surgeon who produces these numbers. Don't just go to that new bariatric surgeon in your neighborhood; he might have done only a few cases. You need to go to someone who has done a few *hundred* cases, preferably a few thousand, in order to be confident about the outcome. Overall, however, this method is very effective for losing a lot of weight quickly. Patients can typically go home two to three days after surgery and can return to work one to two weeks later if there were no complications.

OPTION 2: GASTRIC SLEEVE

The idea behind this procedure is similar to the Roux-en-Y gastric procedure—the goal is to reduce the size of your stomach so you can only hold so much food. The difference is that this procedure does not distort any anatomy. Instead, surgeons perform a linear staple down the middle of the stomach so that more than half is not useful anymore. The rest remains intact, and food can pass through the normal path.

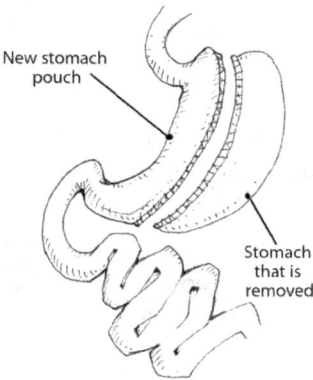

New stomach pouch

Stomach that is removed

Unlike with the Roux-en-Y procedure, the body can continue absorbing all of the nutrients, sugars, and fats as before. Patients do not experience the dumping syndrome as a result of the gastric sleeve procedure. The weight loss is a bit more moderate compared to the rapid weight loss of the Roux-en-Y procedure, however. Patients can expect to lose 40–60 percent of their excess weight in the first year, compared to the 60–80 percent of the other procedure.

The fact that the sleeve does not have many of the same side effects as the Roux-en-Y is attractive to a lot of patients. The procedure is durable, but it's newer than the Roux-en-Y, and leakage can occur if some of the staples ever pop out or move. It is a permanent procedure (irreversible) but can also be used as a bridge to other types of bypass in higher risk patients. The cost is similar to the Roux-en-y gastric procedure and requires the same time in the operating room and similar recovery time. Depending on your BMI, how much weight you need to lose, and how fast you want to get there, this is a procedure to consider. Your surgeon will let you know if you are a good candidate for this method.

OPTION 3: GASTRIC BAND OR ADJUSTABLE GASTRIC BANDING

The gastric band, or adjustable gastric banding procedure, restricts the volume a patient can eat. It is a laparoscopic procedure, meaning that surgeons don't cut open your stomach. The procedure involves making few small incisions in the abdominal wall to accommodate a small video camera and surgical instruments. The surgeons view the procedure on a separate video monitor to give them a better view and access to key structures. The band is an inflatable silicone device that works similarly to a rubber band placed around the top portion of your stomach. The resulting stomach is a small stomach pouch similar to that of the Roux-en-Y procedure except that there is no cutting involved.

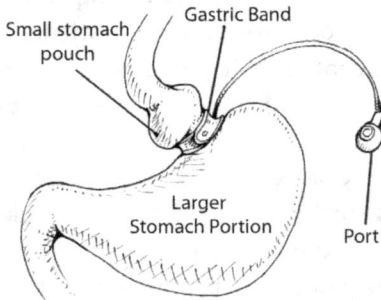

The gastric banding procedure is less complicated than the other two procedures, and people like the fact that it is adjustable and reversible. Patients who are considering having children later can adjust it accordingly so they can lose weight when they need to, increase the size of the stomach before getting pregnant, and then reduce it again later. We believe this to be a durable solution, but since it's a lot newer than the other procedures, we do not have much long-term data to go by.

Patients are often sent home from the hospital within a day of having this procedure and can frequently return to work within a week. However, some people complain that the gastric band does not control their hunger as well as the other two procedures do. Another major complaint with this method is severe nausea and vomiting. Without a doubt, weight loss is slower with this than with the other two methods, but loss is still significant. The exact percentage varies depending on how small your pouch is, your starting weight, etc.; every patient determines how much weight he or she wants to lose, and the surgeon chooses the size of the band depending on those goals. If patients are not meeting the goal, they go in for an adjustment. Adjustments are done without surgery and can take as little as 10 minutes. The process entails a medical professional injecting saline solution into the port and tubing attached to the band.

QUALIFYING AND PREPARING FOR SURGERY

Preparing for bariatric surgery is actually a lengthy process, beginning with a long list of qualifications. First, patients must meet the BMI requirement and be between 18 and 65 years old. Bariatric surgery is not for someone who put on 70 pounds in the last six months; rather, it is for someone who has been carrying excess weight for a good two to five years, and it must be documented for insurance companies to consider paying. Sometimes the insurance company requires the primary care doctors to give them the patient's records showing all of the office visits and weights for the last couple of years.

Insurance companies often put other stipulations on the procedure as well. These might include going on a diet for three to six months in order to document that you can lose some weight on your own. They may require you to lose 10 percent of your body weight before they will approve the procedure. For someone who weighs 300 or 400 pounds, that is *hard!* We're talking about 40 pounds here. That alone could take a year to accomplish for many patients, and it may be the reason they give up on the surgery altogether or are disqualified by the insurance company.

Surgeons also have their own recommendations before they will perform the procedure. They might tell the patient that he must shrink his liver before surgery because the liver is too large due to fat and may be covering the operation site. To shrink the liver, doctors will put the patient on a two-week liquid diet. We talked about how hard liquid diets are; some patients feel as if they are going to die in those two weeks, and some will decide they cannot do it. You also have to stop smoking. Smoking can cause poor healing, so we encourage patients to quit six months before they go into surgery.

When you think of doing bariatric surgery, know that it might be a whole year before you even qualify. It's not as if you can wake up one day and decide, "Oh, I'm 100 pounds overweight—I'm going to see my surgeon!" You have to plan ahead. It takes time before the insurance company will qualify you and more time before you find the surgeon with whom you feel comfortable. You have to do your own research. Then there is medical clearance, which means you might have to undergo stress tests that make sure your heart will withstand the procedure. There is also a battery of pre-op tests that check things like vitamin levels and the thyroid; and you may need an ultrasound, endoscopy, bone scan, blood checks, X-rays, and other procedures before you'll be given the green light. On top of that, be prepared to see a dietician, a social worker, a psychiatrist for counseling, the nurse, the surgeon, and a primary care doctor in order to coordinate everything that's needed. All this before the surgery! Exhausting to think about, isn't it?

I will tell you this: bariatric surgery is not a process for the weak. You have to focus on the fact that you really want this—your health and your life depend on its success. There are also support groups for bariatric surgery, both within bariatric centers and online. Patients often find that support is crucial to getting through the intense waiting period of qualification and preparation.

COMPLICATIONS AND LIFE AFTER BARIATRIC SURGERY
Patients who undergo bariatric surgery must adopt a whole new way of life. They'll eat a very specific, modified diet and will require supplements. They'll need to exercise to strengthen joints and muscles. They must avoid anti-inflammatory medicines like Ibuprofen, aspirin or Aleve, which can cause stomach ulcers. They must avoid taking diuretics, because it can cause electrolyte problems—and if a patient is already not getting enough electrolytes because of the new diet, she doesn't want to take a medicine that is now going to deplete the little she does have.

Once you undergo bariatric surgery, you are married to your surgeon—so make sure you find one you like! You'll see him or her at least five or six times per year for two years to make sure there are no complications, and then less after that. If you opt for gastric banding, you see your surgeon even more often, because they sometimes need to adjust the band to help you lost weight faster or slower.

After any bariatric procedure, it's often a shock for patients to discover how little food or fluid their new stomach can hold. Exactly how much is one ounce? Two or three French fries can fill up a stomach that size, so when we say you cut back on the amount of food you can eat, we really mean it! It will change the way you eat for the rest of your life. You cannot eat and drink at the same time. You must plan ahead since your stomach can only hold a small amount. A patient who is constantly eating may be lucky to consume around 800–1,000 calories a day. Most will never be able to return to a 2,000-calorie diet.

Though the calorie count is low, we don't believe your body goes into starvation mode (burning muscle for energy) after these surgeries. We don't see the visual symptoms that go along with this condition, unless the patient is not consistently taking protein and vitamin supplements. Also, once you have these procedures done, you are no longer on a diet that is restricting you from eating; you can munch every two hours if you want to. You just can't gorge on an entire plate of food anymore. It won't go down.

Keep in mind that bariatric procedures aiding weight loss also lead to better health. Diabetes often improves or disappears, and blood pressure and cholesterol lower. For some, sleep apnea improves, arthritis pain lessens, and stress urinary incontinence gets better. For those who have been taking 10 different medications a day for obesity-related conditions, these weight loss procedures can be a miracle. That's why more insurance companies are falling in line to pay (albeit after the qualification process)—because they see the benefit for patients over a lifetime and know they can ultimately save money by treating them with this one surgery.

The complications arising from these surgeries, however, are not small. There are immediate complications as well as long-term complications. Immediate complications include tissue injury—while the surgeon is in there snipping, stapling, and sewing, he can accidentally poke through the liver, spleen, stomach, esophagus, pancreas, blood vessels, or nerves. There is risk of infection every time your skin is cut into, as well as risk of bleeding or needing transfusions, heart impact from the surgery and anesthesia, and/or organ failure. Things happen. Going to a good surgeon in a center of excellence known for these procedures helps reduce some of these risks.

Things like bowel obstruction can also happen because the bowels are moved during surgery. The bowels are a *really* long tube, and it is all wrapped in there neatly and nicely. When we go in and move things around, putting objects where they weren't before, obstruction can develop if bowels get twisted on themselves. Bowel obstruction causes severe nausea, vomiting, and abdominal pain. Often, patients can't hold anything down, and they have to be admitted to the hospital to prevent dehydration.

Sometimes, the small pouch that was created by the surgery suffers even further narrowing. When we cut through the bowel, inflammation happens, and the body tries to heal. The inflammation can make the pouch narrower or smaller, causing reflux, nausea, and other related symptoms. Stomach ulcers have also been reported, so many patients are placed on medications to prevent this.

Gallstone formation is a common complication of bariatric surgery due to rapid fat loss. Excess bile acids are made to try to break down the fat, but huge quantities just end up forming gallstones, which causes obstruction of the ducts, severe abdominal pain, and infection. Many surgeons now simply plan to take the gallbladder out while they are in the operating room for the weight loss surgery to help avoid this common complication.

Patients can also suffer from inflammation called gout. This causes pain in joints such as the big toe, knees, elbow, and wrist. It is due to increased uric acid levels during rapid weight loss.

Other complications can include leakage from stitched and stapled sites. (We call those anastomotic leaks). This may be because you need an extra stitch somewhere, something got stretched, or a staple fell out. Your surgeon will repair this if found.

Sometimes, with the gastric band surgery, the band can slip or erode into the stomach, allowing the stomach to become large again. There have also been a few cases of allergic reaction to the band material since the body can always react negatively to any foreign material, no matter how good or durable the material is.

Another common and actually expected complication of bariatric surgery is loose skin; you lose weight rapidly and are left with areas of loose skin. Many patients end up needing a second surgery—usually on the excess skin around the stomach area called pannus. Resection is cosmetic, similar to a tummy tuck. Depending on its size, cutting it out can help a patient drop up to another 10 pounds.

Psychosocial issues are another post-surgery complication. Many patients have been dealing with issues stemming from obesity for a long time. Now, when they rapidly lose all that weight, depression can be even more severe. Self-image issues don't away go away with surgery either. They might experience hair loss and have a hard time adapting. For some patients, the issues that caused the weight gain in the first place, such as emotional eating, still have to be dealt with, and because they can no longer use food as comfort, we'll see patients trading addictions; instead of food, they reach for cigarettes or alcohol. The divorce rate is also relatively higher in the post-bariatric weight loss patients than in the general population. Patients are dealing with complex emotions—Johnny accepted her the way she was before, but now that she's lost weight, she's too good for him. Tension is created in relationships, and patients need help to work through it. These are some of the reasons patients must go through a psychosocial evaluation from a psychiatrist prior to surgery.

Follow-ups are also required and extremely important. To be a successful lifetime bariatric patient, you have to be compliant. You have to take your meds, follow up with your appointments, and let your surgeon know if you're experiencing any complications. You must be proactive and involved with your doctors so that anything I've listed can be caught early and taken care of.

Despite the fear factor of these cautions, everything goes the way that textbooks say it should with 85 percent of bariatric surgery patients. Another 10 to 15 percent have transient problems—maybe a little leakage or some nausea, vomiting or diarrhea. Another one percent will have severe complications, where they experience serious health problems or even death. Patients should be aware of this when considering bariatric weight loss options because there is not a guaranteed smooth course for everyone. Before you opt for bariatric surgery, make sure you've put in your best effort and you've tried everything ... including my secret weapon.

CHAPTER 10

MY SECRET WEAPON:
HGC DIET PROTOCOL

AS you know, I didn't always have a weight management issue, and I vowed I would not struggle with it for the rest of my life. After much trial and error with *many* weight loss methods, I can tell you exactly how I regained control: the HCG Diet Protocol.

DISCOVERING THE SECRET WEAPON

I heard of HCG—human chorionic gonadotropin—being used as an injectable weight loss method long before I ever used it. Back then, I didn't pay much attention to the concept because I did not have a weight problem. It wasn't personal yet. I was still under the old school impression that if you wanted to lose weight, you just needed to eat less and exercise more. (So naive, right?) At one time, I remember seeing a billboard sign advertising Lose 1 pound a day with HCG! Of course, I thought it was yet another weight loss gimmick.

It would be a good seven years before my own diet and exercise regimen was failing me and I had 40 pounds to lose. Then I began doing my research and came across the HCG method again.

HCG is a glycoprotein hormone, normally secreted by cells of the placenta in pregnant women. It is somewhat similar in structure to three other pituitary gland hormones: LH (luteinising hormone), FSH (follicle stimulating hormone) and TSH (thyroid stimulating hormone). All four hormones have a protein structure that contains two separate units called alpha and beta chains bound together. All four hormones have nearly identical alpha chains suggesting that they can interact with similar, if not the same, receptors in the body. Their beta units are all different, which is what gives each one its own unique functional properties. While LH and FSH work on the male and female reproductive systems, TSH works on the thyroid gland. HCG, on the other hand, works on the hypothalamus in the brain to affect fat metabolism. HCG can also be used, at high doses, to perform some of the function of LH in patients with infertility issues because of these structural similarities.

I first read about the HCG Diet Protocol in an article on obesity and weight loss in a medical journal called *The Lancet*. I briefly scanned the abstract and saw the acronym "HCG." The only thing I knew about HCG at the time was that it is the hormone in the urine that we test to find out if a woman is pregnant. Besides that one billboard, I never really heard anyone talk about it much, not even in medical school or residency. The few doctors I later found out who knew about it viewed it as an alternative weight loss method and didn't spent much time educating themselves about its use as an obesity treatment. But the more I researched, the more piqued my curiosity became!

I remember typing "HCG" and "weight loss" into Google, and up popped all this data. I saw before and after pictures of people who had used it as a weight loss method. I read reviews and testimonials about the diet. People were saying they had taken everything out there and tried every diet without success, but that the HCG plan really worked for them. They reported eating a very low 500-calorie diet with the injectable medication and all swore they were *not* hungry or starving. Most said they were losing half a pound to a pound every day and remained quite energetic. After my long, unsuccessful struggle to lose my excess pounds, this seemed too good to be true. I wanted to know more and needed to find out if it would work for me.

I went back into the medical journals for more science-based explanations. My research took me as far back as articles from the 1950s and 1970s. I noticed there were no significant harmful effects of HCG injections described or reported in medical literature from that time to today (well over 60 years!). On top of that, I scoured more recent information—medically conducted clinical trials, weight loss journey blogs, before and after pictures, YouTube video logs of thousands of people on HCG—and noted that patients on the protocol did not look emaciated, as someone in "starvation mode" would. Their testimonies were consistent with the very first research protocol using HCG. How was this even possible?

THE HISTORY AND SCIENCE OF THE HCG PROTOCOL

When HCG was first discovered by Ascheim and Zondek in 1927, they found out that it matured the infant sex glands of experimental animals and that it was also secreted by the human placenta. That's where it got the name human chorionic (to relay the placenta) gonadotropin (relating to sex organ). Back then, HCG had to be extracted from the urine of pregnant women, but nowadays most is genetically engineered.

The original study on the effects of HCG as a weight loss method was first reported in 1954 by Dr. Albert T.W. Simeons, a British endocrinologist whose clinic was in Ospedale Salvatori Mundii International Hospital, in Rome, Italy. Wanting to know as much as I could, I read everything ever published by and about Dr. Simeons.

He was born in London and graduated summa cum laude in medicine at the University of Heidelberg. After postgraduate studies in Germany and Switzerland, he became engrossed in the study of tropical diseases and joined the School of Tropical Medicine in Hamburg. He went to India in 1930 while trying to find cures for diseases such as malaria. In 1931, he was awarded the Red Cross Order of Merit by the Queen of England for his injection remedy for malaria and a method of staining malaria parasites, which is known as "Simeons' Stain."

While in India, Dr. Simeons got involved in treating a group of teenage boys called "the fat boys" because they had an endocrine disorder that delayed puberty and made them extremely obese. While treating their undescended testes with HCG, Dr. Simeons observed that the fat boys' body fat distribution changed for the better during treatment. He theorized that if those boys ate a very low calorie diet while on the HCG, they might just start reducing their body weight as well. When he tried it, that was exactly what happened. He then hypothesized that HCG must be acting at the hypothalamus regulatory centers, which is the weight control center in the brain responsible for how much excessive fat is accumulated in the body. He believed that HCG works through the hypothalamus to consequently affect abnormal fat tissue metabolism.

Later, while still stationed in India, Dr. Simeons observed that many pregnant Indian women, although malnourished and severely underweight, gave birth to healthy, normal height, robust babies. He could not understand how the babies could be so healthy when their mothers were so undernourished. This was somewhat of a medical oxymoron for Dr. Simeons, who felt these babies should also be malnourished. He also discovered that obese pregnant women lost weight if they did not overeat or stuff themselves thinking they were "eating for two" during their pregnancy. His curiosity led him to discover that since a pregnant woman's placenta produces HCG, it must be responsible for the mobilization of the excess fat in these women to provide constant free-flowing nutrients to their growing fetuses. Dr. Simeons wrote, "In pregnancy it would be most undesirable if the fetus were offered ample food only when there is a high influx from the intestinal tract. Ideal nutritional conditions for the fetus can only be achieved when the mother's blood is continually saturated with food, regardless of whether she eats or not, as otherwise a period of starvation might hamper the steady growth of the embryo."

A non-pregnant woman does not have the hormone HCG; it is the placenta's job to supply nutrients to the baby, and the placenta is what actually secretes this hormone. Dr. Simeons hypothesized that the production of HCG must have something to do with supplying calories to the fetus to keep up with its constant growth and development. And he concluded that this was of great importance, since the mother was obviously not eating constantly or could be nauseous and unable to keep food down during the first trimester or even longer. The first trimester, he noted, is a critical time in the development of the fetus, because the fetus grows the fastest at this point and needs an uninterrupted supply of calories. Based on his observations, he supposed that the HCG was burning fat from the mother and using it as energy for the baby.

THE WEIGHT SET POINT

The hypothalamus is the part of the brain that controls things such as metabolism, autonomic nervous system, appetite, hunger, thirst, sleep, mood, and weight, among many other functions. Dr. Simeons figured that this hormone, HCG, has a structure that allows it to interact with the hypothalamus, causing it to send signals to decrease hunger and increase fat cell metabolism. He also concluded that HCG doesn't only affect your fat cells; it "talks" to the hypothalamus to change your set weight. There is a premise called the set-point theory, which states that there is a control system built into every person, almost like a thermostat, dictating how much fat or weight he or she should carry. For some, it is set high; for others low. The theory was originally developed in 1982 by Bennett and Gurin to explain why repeated dieting is unsuccessful in producing long-term change in body weight or shape. Going on a weight loss diet attempts to alter the set point by lowering it, but the set point is an untiring opponent ready to undo any such change.

According to the theory, the set point itself keeps weight fairly constant by making the conscious mind change its behavior, feelings, hunger, and/or satiety level. We start our diet at a certain set point, and after an initial, relatively quick loss, we often become stuck at a plateau and then lose weight at a much slower rate. When the set point is driven too low by dieting, the body reacts as though famine has come. It tries to conserve calories by holding more tightly to its fat stores; this is an inborn biological process at work.

The ideal approach to permanent weight loss, then, would have to be a safe method that lowers the set point permanently rather than simply altering it. So far, regular exercise is the most capable activity that we know can lower the set point successfully. Dr Simeons' protocol however, also suggests that HCG affects this set point by interacting with the hypothalamus gland, which is the proposed home of the set point thermostat.

All of this was theory—Dr. Simeons did not know for certain whether HCG could be successfully used as a weight loss method when he set out. The only way to find out would be to give the same hormones to a person who was overweight or had excess body fat to see whether it worked similarly as it did in pregnant women and the fat boys. He believed that if it did, the freely available abnormal excess fat under HCG must be consumed as energy for weight to be lost. This could only be accomplished by combining the HCG injections with restricted calorie intake.

Obviously, Dr. Simeons had a lot to figure out—how much hormone to use, best formulation (tablet, powder, liquid, spray, cream, etc.), the best method of delivery (oral, injection, intramuscular, intravenous, subcutaneous, sublingual, etc.), and so on. He also needed to determine how many calories should be consumed for the diet, what food groups to include or eliminate, how many meals per day, how much and what to drink ... After much practice (trial and error), he found that by using a tiny dose of 125 units as a daily injection, he got consistent results. To put the dosage in perspective, a pregnant woman might have up to a million units of HCG in her body at any one point. But only 125 units of HCG, combined with a specific 500-calorie low-carb, low-fat, lean protein diet, was effective.

He later extended his investigations to patients showing different degrees of obesity. For 16 years in his clinic in Rome, he worked on perfecting his weight loss theory of how low daily doses of HCG injections combined with an ultra-low-calorie diet quickly encourage the loss of fat with no consequential muscle loss. In that time, he successfully treated over 10,000 patients, many of whom were royalty or wealthy enough to spend a minimum of 40 days, or the entire treatment course, in his clinic in Rome. He concluded that HCG might be more useful for the treatment of obesity than the medical community ever thought. Dr. Simeons found, as added benefits, that his patients had no headaches, hunger pains, weakness, or irritability, which are normally seen in ultra low caloric diets. His method also helped to naturally reshape the patients' bodies even if they did not engage in exercise while on the protocol. Dr. Simeons concluded that this was because the patients were only losing excess fat, which made their real body shape more visible.

So, in 1954, Dr. Simeons published the book, *Pounds and Inches: A New Approach to Obesity*. This book gives the exact protocol that he used in his clinic. Today, HCG is still recognized by many weight loss clinics for its abilities to help patients lose dramatic amounts of fat weight. Although

HCG is not approved by the FDA as a weight loss treatment, the FDA has determined that it is safe to use.

As my research became more involved, I had to process all this new information as a doctor. First, I realized that this protocol was coming from an endocrinologist—someone who not only studied internal medicine like myself but also specialized for an additional three years in fellowship training to better understand how hormones function. I got the idea of HCG causing release of excess body fat but asked myself why we couldn't just eat anything we wanted while on the HCG protocol. Why did we have to go on such a restricted diet? My reasoning was that if I continued to consume my 2,200 calories per day, my body— which preferred lazy sugars and carbs for energy—would rather use those than work to burn the excess fat it had spent a lot of energy to store away. Therefore, the fat that HCG worked hard to release would just float around until the body stashed it away again. By restricting the amount of food I took in, my body was forced to get the rest of the energy it needed for daily functioning from somewhere else; *that* is how I began to see excess fat loss.

As I've touched on, one of my major concerns with what the FDA has to offer in terms of weight loss drugs are the side effects. With HCG, I was not worried about that. In over 60 years since Dr. Simeons' original research was done, there have been no adverse reports from people who have used it—not one single report of side effects since the 1950s. In terms of safety profile, HCG has a clean record. I also decided that any medicine or hormone that is safe in the presence of a fetus for several months was probably safe for me to use.

As I dug more into the medical history of Dr. Simeons' study, I found additional studies confirming his theories and findings. Of course, I also came across other studies that claimed Dr. Simeon's theory was incorrect and that his plan did not work, but some of those also did not always follow his protocol in its entirety. Those that did were successful. At that point, I made a bold—and controversial—choice: I would try HCG.

MY PERSONAL SUCCESS STORY

I decided to inquire about the process through a free consultation from a doctor-monitored clinic, rather than prescribing HCG to myself or going to just any weight loss clinic that happened to offer HCG. The reason I went this route is because Dr. Simeons said that HCG required close physician monitoring. In fact, he only treated patients who were willing to spend the entire 40 days at his clinic in Rome.

The clinic I chose was very modern, elegant, and inviting, unlike the classic sterile doctor's office. It had a nurturing, yet professional, look. The waiting room was not overloaded, and they actually kept to my appointment time (imagine that). I didn't tell anyone at the clinic that I was a physician so that I was treated like all its other patients.

Before I stepped barefoot on the body analyzer scale, I had to remove all metals—my earrings, watch, and belt. The scale sent small electrodes through my body to calculate my numbers—how much muscle, fat, water, and bone mass I had—as well as my BMI. The scale even broke down how much fat was in specific parts of my body: my hands, my belly, my thighs …

I remember looking at my body composition printout and seeing my percentage of body fat—43.6 percent. My body was nearly half fat! I was shocked. The analysis said that I should weigh 160 pounds for my six foot height, but I was at 230 pounds. Composed of half fat. At the rate I had been losing weight, it was going to take a long time to reach a healthy range.

At my consultation, the doctor performed a physical and drew blood to test whether I had diabetes or cholesterol, liver, or thyroid problems. The doctor was thorough and answered all my questions—and let me tell you, I put him through the ringer! I wanted to make sure he was at the top of his game before I underwent any sort of procedure under his guidance.

The nurse practitioner explained the process of the HCG diet and shared testimonials of the patients with whom the clinic had worked. She said, "With two rounds of HCG, you can be there. You can lose those excess pounds and be at your ideal weight in no time."

I shook my head in disbelief. Though I'd read the testimonials and heard people sharing their stories, I had been battling my weight and trying to simply lose and keep off 10 pounds for so long. I said, "Lady, you don't know what you're talking about! It took me nearly two years of working hard, training every day, to lose just 10 pounds. And now you're telling me that I can lose 60 pounds or more in three months?" It was mind-boggling. She answered by telling me her own personal experience. She was a really slim, tall woman, so I never even guessed that she might have needed the protocol herself at some point. However, she had lost 30 pounds in just six weeks and had kept it off for over two years. Wow! I started becoming more convinced it might work for me, too.

Despite the research I'd already done, I decided I wanted and needed to learn more before I went ahead with this diet plan myself. I poured over the online video logs and side effects patients said they were experiencing, but I noted they were nothing serious—maybe some mild headaches during the first few days, or some fatigue, but they all confirmed it went away by the end of the first week. The best part was that they were all consistently losing weight. Some patients reported a stall in their weight loss by the fourth or fifth week, meaning they weren't losing pounds, but they tended to lose inches on those days. I decided it was worth a shot. I went back to the clinic with the mindset that I did not have anything to lose—except the excess weight, of course.

By the time I returned to the clinic and enrolled, my starting weight was 230 pounds. After my lab work came back, I took the first step in my HCG journey. The clinic showed me how to give myself the HCG injection and how to begin the program. I began the HCG diet protocol and I stuck to it. I did feel a little hungry with a mild headache for the first couple of days, but by the third day on the diet, I was no longer hungry and the headache was gone. I didn't feel tired, and I didn't feel weak. I actually had a lot of energy and was able to continue with my day-to-day routine and functions without a hitch. I was working in the hospital on 25 patients a day and going up and down flights of stairs, rushing to the emergency room and medical wards, and I was fine. I knew I had to be surviving on more than just the 500 calories I was consuming for me to do all that work without problems. But the magic was *really* confirmed every morning: when I woke up and weighed myself, I had lost anywhere from a half a pound to one pound from the day before. This was my motivation to continue on the protocol without cheating. And at the end of the 40 days, I had lost a total of 30 pounds. Me? Thirty pounds gone forever? I was ecstatic.

THE HCG DIET

In order for the HCG protocol to work, I needed to follow the exact diet Dr. Simeons laid out in his original protocol. It goes as follows:

Breakfast:
Water, tea, or coffee without sugar. Only one tablespoon of milk allowed in 24 hours.

Lunch:
- 100 grams of veal, beef, chicken breast, fresh white fish, lobster, crab, or shrimp, boiled or grilled without additional fat. Remove all visible fat before cooking.
- Salmon, eel, tuna, herring, dried or pickled fish are not allowed.
- Choose one vegetable (usually about three cups) from the following: spinach, chard, chicory, beet-greens, green salad, tomatoes, celery, fennel, onions, red radishes, cucumbers, asparagus, or cabbage.
- One breadstick (grissini) or one Melba toast.
- One apple, a medium orange, a handful of strawberries (about eight), or half a grapefruit.

Dinner:
Same choices as lunch.

Other important tips:

1 The 500-calorie limit must always be maintained.

2 Tea, coffee, plain water, or mineral water (two liters of water per day is recommended) are allowed and may be taken in any quantity and at all times.

3 The juice of one lemon daily is allowed for all purposes.

4 Salt, pepper, vinegar, mustard powder, garlic, sweet basil, parsley, thyme, marjoram, etc., may be used for seasoning but no oil, butter or dressing.

5 The fruit or the breadstick may be eaten between meals instead of with lunch or dinner if desired.

6 Occasionally we allow eggs—boiled, poached, or raw— to patients who develop an aversion to meat, but in this case they must add the whites of three eggs to the one they eat whole.

7 Cottage cheese made from skim milk is allowable; 100 grams may occasionally be used instead of the meat.

8 No medicines or cosmetics other than lipstick, eyebrow pencil, and powder may be used without special permission. However, aspirin and birth control are allowed.

9 No massages of any kind are allowed because it disturbs a very delicate process going on in the tissues. Thumping, rolling, or kneading only results in severe bruising, tissue tearing, scar formation, and harder and more unyielding fat tissue.

DAYS 1–2

The first two days of protocol are gorge days, meaning you eat anything and everything you want. It's all fair game: high-fat, high-sugar, high-carb foods—you are supposed to load up for the first two days, and load up I did! I ate everything I love—Breyers Vanilla Bean Ice Cream, a large-portioned meal at The Cheesecake Factory, bagels, fried chicken. I ate like crazy! The reason for the two gorge days, according to Dr Simeons, is:

> "One cannot keep a patient comfortably on 500 calories unless his normal fat reserves are reasonably well stocked. It is for this reason also that every case, even those that are actually gaining, must eat to capacity of the most fattening food they can get down until they have had the third injection. It is a fundamental mistake to put a patient on 500 calories as soon as the injections are started, as it seems to take about three injections before abnormally deposited fat begins to circulate and thus become available."

Honestly, by the end of those two days, I was ready for the diet to begin. I was sick of eating, I didn't want to see another fatty food near me, and I was stuffed. As for the injection, it was not painful at all. The clinic used the smallest insulin needles possible. I cleaned my belly area with an alcohol swab and injected into the fat under my skin. There was no pain (just a minor flinch), no bruising, no bleeding; nothing.

DAYS 3–40

After the two loading days, I began the 500-calorie diet. Before day three, I went to the grocery store and bought all of my allowed meats. I asked the butcher to cut the meat into 100-gram servings just like the protocol required. I ordered fish, chicken, and lean beef; because it was already portioned, all I had to do was season it and throw it on the grill or in the oven. I bought the allowed fresh vegetables, and I stocked up on Honeycrisp apples—my favorite! And since Dr. Simeons did not specify the size of the apples, I loaded up on the biggest ones I could find! (He does specify only half of a grapefruit at a time.) I also bought strawberries and oranges.

The first day on the 500-calorie diet, I had a mild headache, similar to those I usually get when I'm hungry. The amazing thing was that, after I ate my meal, the headache went away—no medication required, as it usually is for me.

The next day, I had some mild discomfort, but I can't even call it a headache. It, too, disappeared after eating.

By the third day, I was not feeling any hunger or headache. I had energy and was coasting through.

Day four was when I saw my first weight loss: over three pounds. Three pounds!

By day five, I'd lost another two pounds. I thought, *Wow! If I continue at this rate, I'll lose 80 pounds in 40 days!*

After the fifth day, I lost anywhere from half a pound to a pound a day. I've included my personal log below so that you can see my astonishing progress.

HCG Round 1   Page 1/2

▶ TAKE "BEFORE" PHOTO!

9/29 (date) START	9/30	10/1 TRAINING BLOCK	10/2 1	10/3	10/4	10/5
DIET Y (N) 1	DIET Y (N) 2	DIET Y N 3	DIET Y N 4	DIET Y N 5	DIET Y N 6	DIET Y N 7
231.2	232.4	233.6	230.2	228.0	226.0	224.2
Loading day	Loading day	Day 1 of diet				

10/6	10/7	10/8	10/9	10/10	10/11	10/12
DIET Y N 8	DIET Y N 9	DIET Y N 10	DIET Y N 11	DIET Y N 12	DIET Y N 13	DIET Y N 14
223.0	222.4	221.2	220.2	219.2	219.0	218.6
				TOM	TOM*	TOM*

10/13	10/14	10/15	10/16	10/17	10/18	10/19
DIET Y N 15	DIET Y N 16	DIET Y N 17	DIET Y N 18	DIET Y N 19	DIET Y N 20	DIET Y N 21
218.2	217.8	216.8	215.8	215.3	214.8	214.3
TOM*	TOM*					

10/20	10/21	10/22	10/23	10/24	10/25	10/26
DIET Y N 22	DIET Y N 23	DIET Y N 24	DIET Y N 25	DIET Y N 26	DIET Y N 27	MEASURE BODY FAT % TAKE ◀ PHOTO! 28
214.3	214.0	214.2	213.2	212.6	212.0	211.6
WNS**	WNS**	WNS**				

NOTES

* TOM = Time of Month (women's menstral period)
** WNS = Worked Night Shift   **DECIDE**

🔵 BEACHBODY

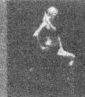

FOR SUPPORT AND TIPS AND TO BUILD ON YOUR SUCCESS, VISIT **Beachbody.com/P90X,** OR

I woke at the same time every day, emptied my bladder, weighed myself, gave myself my injection, and then drank my tea, coffee, or water, and went about my day.

I remember first seeing my family when I went home for a visit. I had about a week left of protocol. By this point, I had lost about 20 pounds, and when they saw me, they said, "Wow! Look at you! You look great!" I told them about my 500-calorie diet, and they were shocked by the low number. But, they added, it was obviously working for me, so they encouraged me to keep it up. And I did.

HCG   Round 1   Page ²/2

▶ TAKE "BEFORE" PHOTO!

10/27 START	10/28	10/29 TRAINING BLOCK	10/30 2	10/31	11/1	11/2
DIET Y N 1	DIET Y N 2	DIET Y N 3	DIET Y N 4	DIET Y N 5	DIET Y N 6	DIET Y N 7
211.1	211.1	211.0	210.0	209.0	208.0	207.2
Stall	Stall	Apple Day***				

11/3	11/4	11/5	11/6	11/7	11/8	11/9
DIET Y N 8	DIET Y N 9	DIET Y N 10	DIET Y N 11	DIET Y N 12	DIET Y N 13	DIET Y N 14
206.6	206.2	205.6	203.6	202.4	201.6	200.2
						Last injection

11/10	11/11	11/12	11/13	11/14	11/15	11/16
DIET Y N 15	DIET Y N 16	DIET Y N 17	DIET Y N 18	DIET Y N 19	DIET Y N 20	DIET Y N 21

← ——— out of town   for   Caleb's Birthday →
← ——— on NOV   11th. ———————————→

11/17						
DIET Y N 22	DIET Y N 23	DIET Y N 24	DIET Y N 25	DIET Y N 26	DIET Y N 27	DIET Y N 28
200.2						MEASURE BODY FAT % TAKE ◀ PHOTO!

NOTES

*** Apple Day: ate only 6 apples to break the stall.

DECIDE

⊘ BEACHBODY®

Stabilization   Phase 1/2

NO Carbs, Eating 2000 Calories/day
Increase Exercise

▶ TAKE "BEFORE" PHOTO!

11/10 START	11/11	11/12 TRAINING BLOCK	11/13 1	11/14	11/15	11/16
DIET Y N 1	DIET Y N 2	DIET Y N 3	DIET Y N 4	DIET Y N 5	DIET Y N 6	DIET Y N 7

⇐ Didn't weigh, was out of town ⇒

11/17	11/18	11/19	11/20	11/21	11/22	11/23
DIET Y N 8	DIET Y N 9	DIET Y N 10	DIET Y N 11	DIET Y N 12	DIET Y N 13	DIET Y N 14
200.2	200.2	198.6	197.2	196.4	196.0	195.6
	ELT*	P90X**	ELT*	P90X**	ELT*	Thanksgiving weekend

11/24	11/25	11/26	11/27	11/28	11/29	11/30
DIET Y N 15	DIET Y N 16	DIET Y N 17	DIET Y N 18	DIET Y N 19	DIET Y N 20	DIET Y N 21
195.6	195.0	194.4	193.4	192.9	192.0	190.8
Thanksgiving weekend	P90X** Thanksgiving Day.	ELT*	P90X**	ELT*	P90X**	← lost almost 10 lbs on my own without HCG

DIET Y N 22	DIET Y N 23	DIET Y N 24	DIET Y N 25	DIET Y N 26	DIET Y N 27	DIET Y N 28
						MEASURE BODY FAT % TAKE ◀ PHOTO!

NOTES

*ELT = Eliptical Machine Exercise for at least 1 hr
burning 400 Calories.
** P90X = Ab exercises, Arms & back.
muscle strenghtening

DECIDE

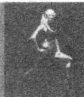

Stabilization   phase 2/2

Start carbs slow.   2200 calories/day

▶ TAKE "BEFORE" PHOTO!

11/31 START	12/1	12/2 TRAINING BLOCK	12/3	12/4	12/5	12/6
DIET Y N *1*	DIET Y N *2*	DIET Y N *3*	DIET Y N *4*	DIET Y N *5*	DIET Y N *6*	DIET Y N *7*
190.0	190.0	193.0	190.0	192.1	190.0	190.0
	ate white rice	Correction Steak Day	ate white Bread	Correction Steak day	ate wheat bread	ate Brown rice
12/7	12/8	12/9	12/10	12/11	12/12	12/13
DIET Y N *8*	DIET Y N *9*	DIET Y N *10*	DIET Y N *11*	DIET Y N *12*	DIET Y N *13*	DIET Y N *14*
190.0	191.3	193.3	190.0	191.8	191.8	193.8
ate Baked Potato	ate Homemade cookies	Correction steak day	ate French fries	ate wheat Crackers	ate pasta (white)	Correction steak day
12/14	12/15	12/16	12/17	12/18	12/19	12/20
DIET Y N *15*	DIET Y N *16*	DIET Y N *17*	DIET Y N *18*	DIET Y N *19*	DIET Y N *20*	DIET Y N *21*
190.2	190.0	192.1	190.0	192.2	190.2	191.2
ate whole grain bread	ate Blueberry Waffle	Correction steak day	ate Potato chips	Correction Steak day	Jelly beans Candy	No carbs today
DIET Y N *22*	DIET Y N *23*	DIET Y N *24*	DIET Y N *25*	DIET Y N *26*	DIET Y N *27*	DIET Y N *28*
						MEASURE BODY FAT %
						TAKE ◀ PHOTO!

NOTES

Exercised every other day for about 50 mins.
(30 mins on Elliptical, 20 mins
      with weights)   **DECIDE**

HCG Round 2   Page 1/1

Exercised Every other day for 50 mins

▶ TAKE "BEFORE" PHOTO!

12/21 START DIET Y N 1	12/22 DIET Y N 2	12/23 DIET Y N 3	12/24 TRAINING BLOCK 1 DIET Y N 4	12/25 DIET Y N 5	12/26 DIET Y N 6	12/27 DIET Y N 7
190.0 Loading day	192.0 Loading day	192.2 Day 1 of Diet	190.0	189.4 Cheated on Christmas Day	189.4	188.0
12/28 DIET Y N 8	12/29 DIET Y N 9	12/29 DIET Y N 10	12/30 DIET Y N 11	12/31 DIET Y N 12	1/1 DIET Y N 13	1/2 DIET Y N 14
187.1	186.4	186.0	185.4	184.4	183.0 Cheated on New Years	183.6
1/3 DIET Y N 15	1/4 DIET Y N 16	1/5 DIET Y N 17	1/6 DIET Y N 18	1/7 DIET Y N 19	1/8 DIET Y N 20	1/9 DIET Y N 21
182.4	182.2	181.5 TOM	180.8 TOM	180.3 TOM	180.1 TOM	180.1 TOM Last injection
1/10 DIET Y N 22	DIET Y N 23	DIET Y N 24	DIET Y N 25	DIET Y N 26	DIET Y N 27	DIET Y N 28 MEASURE BODY FAT % TAKE PHOTO!
180.0						

NOTES

* TOM = Time of Month (women's Menstral period)

DECIDE

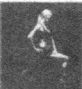

People saw that I was eating less and was on a low-carb diet. I wasn't doing any vigorous exercise during the protocol because the original diet advised against it if your body was not already accustomed to it. So the only exercise I did was an occasional walk with my son around our neighborhood. Still, the weight kept coming off. At the end of those 40 days, I had lost approximately 30 pounds. The word *excited* doesn't begin to cover what I felt!

My original body "set weight" before the protocol must have been around 230, but after completing the diet, it was reset to 180. This reset phenomenon explains why you can get off the HCG and not put the weight back on once you start eating 2,000 calories again. Granted, if you go back to overeating or eating all the wrong foods, then yes, you're going to gain weight—there's no science to that! But more than a month of being on such a diet should have made some changes in you; your choices throughout those 40 days should have become closer to habits. Plus, you *want* to maintain your new weight. You like the way you feel and look, and you revel in compliments from others. This is all motivation to keep up the good behavior.

The HCG process doesn't end there, though.

MAINTENANCE

For the first three weeks after you finish protocol, you are still following a diet of sorts—around 2,000 calories a day and no carbohydrates or simple sugars. To bring my calorie intake up, I increased my portions of protein and ate a lot of vegetables. The goal during these three weeks is to maintain your weight loss while adapting your body to a regular eating routine. I lost 10 additional pounds on my own during this phase because I intensified my exercise and kept to a lean, healthy diet. (See my personal log.)

After that maintenance period, you can start adding in carbs a little at a time. I introduced white rice first because it had been a big part of my diet since I was young. The day after eating half a cup of rice, I gained a few pounds. That let me know it was not good for my body. The next carb I tried was normal servings of white bread with my meals. Another weight gain!

Any time I was up by more than two pounds from my last injection weight, I did what the protocol calls a "steak day," which is designed to correct your weight gain. On a steak day, you start out by fasting, so you don't eat breakfast or lunch. But you are allowed to have steak—any size you want—for dinner, along with an apple or a raw tomato. I thought, *Steak day? I can do this!* And guess what? The extra pounds disappeared by the next day. My body automatically returned to its new set point! That was awesome to see. (Take a look at my personal log.) I admit, I'm not exactly sure how or why this works, but it does, every time. I didn't argue with progress.

The trial and error process told me that I needed to stay away from white rice and white bread, so I began testing different foods to see what was good for my body. I introduced healthier versions of the carbs—brown rice instead of white, whole wheat bread—and my weight remained stable.

By the time those second three weeks of maintenance were done, I was ready to do another round of protocol. Not everyone needs a second round. It is only for those who have more weight to lose. If you do the second round, it has to be a minimum of three weeks but can be as long as six weeks again. I decided to do a shorter version because I only had 10 more pounds to lose. I did a three-week round and lost around half a pound most days. I didn't see the same initial loss as I did on the first round, when I lost two pounds or more at times. However, I was still able to lose 10 pounds without any problems within those three weeks.

Afterwards, I repeated the maintenance phase—three weeks with no sugar or carbs; when I did start introducing carbohydrates again, I took what I learned from my previous experience and stayed away from white rice, white bread, and the like. My weight remained stable, and I didn't need to do a steak day.

Every now and then, I still have some of those "bad carbs," but it is not a daily or even a weekly thing anymore. Mostly, I splurge when I don't have another option, such as when a drug rep brings us lunch or I'm at an event where I need to eat. But by following my diet and using what I've learned, I've been able to keep the weight off and correct any weight gain with a steak day. And let me just say—when I do a steak day, it's a pretty good size steak. I'm talking a large T-bone! And to wake up to a two-pound correction the next day … well, it's hard to believe!

The protocol takes discipline, yes, but my motivation throughout was waking up and knowing that I was going to lose one pound that day. That made me stick to the diet even when we had lunch catered at work or I had to contend with any other function. The one pound I knew I'd lose that day was worth more to me than the cheesecake on the table.

THE CONTROVERSY, THE CRITICS, AND MY REBUTTALS

When colleagues at work saw me shrinking and asked me what I was doing, I told them I was on a low-carb diet. I didn't tell anyone outside my family that it was HCG because I knew about the controversy in the medical community.

A lot of doctors argue that HCG does not work. You're losing weight because you're *starving* yourself, they say, and it's dangerous. But if this is true, and HCG does not work, why aren't individuals on the protocol tired and in starvation mode?

We all know you cannot survive on a 500-calorie diet alone for 40 days. In fact, your body goes into starvation mode with anything less than 800 calories a day. In this state, your body eats its own protein, like your muscle, leaving you feeling weak, tired, and hungry. Your stomach would be growling all the time, you would be irritable, and you would not have energy to go about your daily routine. All you would want to do is lie down somewhere and sleep to conserve energy. You might feel dizzy or lightheaded, and be preoccupied with food.

Also, an individual in starvation mode looks emaciated. And the sad thing for those who intentionally do this to themselves, such as anorexics, is that the body doesn't even try to burn its fat at first. It locks in the fat even more. It's as if the body says, "Okay, we're not getting food here, so we have to save this fat for a real emergency like impending death! Let's use up all this muscle and the glucose in the liver and everything else first, before we even *think* about touching the fat in storage!" So your belly does not go away, you don't look normal, and you start having electrolyte problems. Starvation mode puts the body in a bad state, and I can see why people are concerned that this plan includes a 500-calorie diet.

In the 1940s, experts conducted a study called The Minnesota Starvation Study. In it, able-bodied men—men who were high achieving, well built, and well nourished—from all walks of life were enrolled for six months. During that time, the participants lived in a boot-camp type of setting where they were only allowed to eat half their daily required calories. Researchers monitored their every move, 24 hours a day.

By the end of the six months, most of the participants had lost a quarter of their starting weight. And what researchers noticed was that bizarre things were happening to these men. Prior to the study, the participants were motivated, well-rounded, happy people. Six months later, they were nervous, restless, moody, depressed, distracted, and unable to concentrate. Their interest in life had narrowed, they had lost their ambition, they were easily frustrated and irritable, and some of them became violent. Some even inflicted injury on themselves so they could be dismissed from the camp. They became preoccupied with food, and that was all they talked about. Some of the men removed pictures of their girlfriends from the wall and put pictures of food up instead. They constantly talked about how hungry they were and which foods would really taste good. Their extreme hunger preoccupied them all day long, and when it came to mealtimes, they were licking their plates and fingers. A lot of them even chewed on their hands and nails.

Additionally, researchers noted that the participants' metabolic rates had decreased because their bodies were trying to adjust to the lower amount of calories they were eating. Their pulse, heart rate, and body temperature also lowered, so the men felt cold all the time. Many of them lost muscle, felt weak, and struggled to climb stairs they had no problem with at the beginning of the study. Their skin felt cold and scaly, and its elasticity had decreased. Some of the participants developed brownish pigment in their skin, which is a condition caused from a high level of a hormone called ACTH, which is a stress hormone. Researchers hypothesized that the men's cortisol level was probably high as well. As if that wasn't enough, a lot of the participants developed skin ulcers and cold sores, their libido was down, they experienced dizziness and headaches, and they got muscle cramps when they were sleeping. During physical exams, their reflexes were sluggish, and the men reported feeling "older." Based on this study, we know that these symptoms occur in the human body when it has entered starvation mode. And in this case, the men had only cut their diets down to half their daily required calories—nowhere close to 500.

If you were eating 500 calories a day and were not on HCG, your body could potentially have enough glycogen stores for three days. (Glycogen is used as an emergency glucose when you're not eating and your body needs it—for example, when you're working out.) But within a week, you would begin experiencing some of symptoms the men in the study struggled with—*none* of which have ever been reported by patients on the HCG protocol. Including me.

The funny thing is, by week two, most HCG patients report they are feeling their best! They are coasting through the diet and aren't hungry anymore. They are experiencing no headaches, have plenty of energy, and start asking if they can skip some meals because they actually feel full! I tell them they *must* eat those meals and have all their 500 calories.

Critics need to understand the science behind the HCG diet protocol. Yes, you are consuming only 500 calories a day, but if your body is burning the excess and abnormal fat you have stored, it is making up for the remaining 1,500 or more calories it needs. The people who argue against the HCG method are not looking at the fact that the body is getting those extra calories from your fat stores. In a way, you *are* consuming 2,000 calories a day while on the HCG diet protocol! I wonder what these critics would say to the people who have experienced success or to my patients, who don't feel like they are in starvation mode, are able to do their daily functions, and aren't hungry, cranky, or weak. What do the critics say to these people who are thriving on the diet? What do they say to weekly body composition analysis reports that show patients' muscle mass is stable and fat percentage is going down?

There are other arguments staring critics in the face as well. The liver of the HCG patient, for instance, looks better than it did before. Diabetic numbers improve, so much so that I am taking patients off their insulin! I am cutting their blood pressure medicine in half or discontinuing it. I am taking them off their cholesterol medicine because their numbers are now in normal range. Tell me how a starvation mode diet does all of that!

Are you curious about the FDA's stance on HCG? My research shows that the FDA has approved HCG for three things only, all to do with fertility and hypergonadism. They do not have any negative reports of this medication in terms of effects, but they also have not approved it for weight loss. Their position is that if physicians decide to use HCG for weight loss, they must offer a disclaimer to the patient saying: "HCG has not been demonstrated to be effective adjunctive therapy in the treatment of obesity. There is no substantial evidence that it increases weight loss beyond that resulting from caloric restriction, that it causes a more attractive or 'normal' distribution of fat, or that it decreases the hunger and discomfort associated with calorie-restricted diets."

Now, everyone is entitled to their opinion, but I believe critics of this diet should do some research and see if it makes sense. The HCG diet protocol made sense to me, and that was why I decided to use it. Like me, there are people who are trying it and experiencing life-changing results. And it would be one thing if I were only seeing results in 80 percent of my patients, but I'm seeing results in 100 percent of them. *Every* patient I have put on the plan loses weight effectively. That's pretty compelling evidence. I'll admit, it's more likely to be effective when supervised medically than not. But care must be taken to go to a physician who has the knowledge and experience using the hormone in weight loss.

OTHER METHODS OF HCG USE

Because the HCG method has been shown to be an effective weight loss solution, the diet industry has gotten a hold of it and is trying to find other formulations that people might find easier to use than injections. For someone worried about injections, drops or a spray or cream might be more enticing.

While I have not seen many clinical trials on other formulations, I have seen reports that other physicians have effectively used a sublingual formula, meaning it is placed under the tongue. In this formula, HCG can be mixed with water-soluble vitamin B12, in which the B12 becomes the carrier that allows the hormone to be absorbed. However, the tongue can only absorb so much at a time, so you must take the HCG twice a day instead of once.

The issue I have with sublingual drops is that the amount of absorption depends on how long you can hold it under your tongue. The recommended time is anywhere from 5–10 minutes. The problem is, we're not sure how quickly the body absorbs the formula. The B12 can sometimes create a tingling sensation that makes it hard to keep under the tongue. A lot of patients can only hold it down for maybe three minutes before swallowing the rest—and whatever you swallow is not used, because it cannot be absorbed from your GI tract. The other issue with drops is transporting the medication. It needs to be kept cold and taken twice a day, which I find slightly inconvenient.

So which method do I recommend? For my patients, I recommend injection. I tell them this is what the clinical trials that I am basing my protocol on have studied. If you feel faint when you see a needle, then I will make you a sublingual version. But so far, even my patient who was most scared of needles was willing to do the injections after I showed her how truly painless it was.

The injections are subcutaneous—you pinch a little bit of skin on your belly area and inject the HCG right under the skin into the fat tissue. (And a lot of us have extra fat tissue there!) The needle is short—about half an inch—and you are not trying to reach the muscle or go for a vein. While I sometimes recommend alternating sides of the belly so you aren't poking the same spot every day, most find the injections to be convenient and painless. No bleeding and no reaction at the injection site for at least 99.9 percent of people. Patients can dispose of the needle either in a sharps box, which they can get from their pharmacy, or I allow my patients to bring them in every week for me to dispose of myself. Easy peasy.

HOMEOPATHIC HCG?

While I approve of the versions and doses of HCG that are regulated by prescription, I have a problem with the "homeopathic" versions popping up on the Internet. For a medication to be called homeopathic, the makers need to claim that it only contains "traces" of the hormone. Traces cannot be 125 units, like Dr. Simeons recommended for this diet to work. Otherwise, the manufacturers would need to report back to the FDA and it would then become a prescription medicine. This means the homeopathic versions might have 10 units of HCG, or even 25 or 50 units, but because it cannot be measured, the user has no idea how much, if any, he or she is actually consuming.

People get varied results using the homeopathic version of HCG—some people say it doesn't work and write all over the Internet that HCG is a fraud. The truth is that their homeopathic drops probably contain too little HCG. And with these drops, you don't know exactly what you're taking, yet you are trying to follow a diet protocol that is very specific. If your drops have little or no HCG in them, you *are* putting yourself in starvation mode! Period.

How can you check to see how much HCG is in your drops? You can't. Even if you place a few drops of the homeopathic drops on a pregnancy test (which tests for the HCG hormone), a positive only means there is *some* HCG in there. It doesn't tell you how many units. But for those who are unsure of the product they're using, doing a test would at least help confirm there is some HCG in the drops.

IS HCG ONLY FOR OBESE PATIENTS?

Most patients lose between 20 and 40 pounds on a round of HCG. But if you have less than 20 pounds to lose, can you still use the HCG method? Yes! What I do with those patients is start them on a shorter round. If you have, say, 15 pounds to lose, three weeks should be all it takes. If you have 5 or 10 pounds to lose, you'd still go on the three-week diet because we've found that it takes that long to help your body stabilize at its new weight. The HCG will stop working when you do not have any more abnormal body fat, so if you lose all the excess fat before the three weeks are up, you'd simply stop seeing weight loss. Your body would still reset its weight.

OTHER BENEFITS OF HCG

A bonus of losing weight with HCG is what we call body reshaping.

Because the HCG works on abnormal body fat, it targets the muffin-top, the excess belly fat, and the cellulite in your hips, buttocks, and thighs. So women and men find that even at a higher weight than their goal, their bodies fit into clothes a whole lot better. Even though I now weigh

180 pounds, many of the clothes I wear are the same ones I reached for when I was 160 pounds. My hips have been curved right, and the excess under the buttocks is gone, so the clothes fit great even though I technically weigh more.

I often tell patients on HCG that the goal is not to get where the textbooks say you should weigh; your goal is to get to what is healthy for you. Many times, the textbook says a patient should weigh about 20 pounds less than what I believe they should after doing a body composition analysis. I have to counsel patients to find a weight goal that I believe will work for them.

Typically, I will look at how many pounds of muscle the patient has and add the amount of pounds of fat that he or she should have. For women, I usually allow between 30 and 60 pounds of fat—so if a woman has 100 pounds of muscle, I will add 30 pounds of fat to it, and then I give another 10 pounds for the weight of organs, bones, and water. Based on these calculations, her goal weight should be around 140 pounds, whereas the recommendation according to my printout is 120 pounds. It's important to know your realistic, healthy weight.

Another benefit of the HCG protocol is that it helps teach you what foods are right for your body. Once the entire protocol is finished, you have a six-week period of stabilization (even if all you did was a three-week protocol). During this time, you avoid carbs or sugars for three weeks but can increase your vegetables and protein; I tell my patients to basically triple what they were eating on the diet if they are not bored to death with it already. As we've already discussed, after the first three weeks, you start introducing carbs and learn what works for your body and what doesn't in the next three weeks. You should weigh yourself every day to see how your body reacts to specific foods; the weight you are using as standard at this point is your weight on the last day you injected HCG.

Once you know how different foods affect your weight, you have a good idea of which ones to avoid for the most part. There is nothing off limits, and there is nothing you cannot eat for the rest of your life, but you are more aware of what you're eating and how it affects your body. This learning process helps you stabilize your weight for the long term.

Many people who have been overweight for a long time worry about having saggy skin once they lose the weight. This is what we see in many bariatric patients who undergo weight loss surgery. This is not what we see with HCG. The elasticity in the skin for these dieters is amazing. Don't believe me? Search for "slimsteve503" on YouTube. He lost 100 pounds on this diet, and his skin looks fantastic. I believe the HCG hormone helps your skin retain its elasticity, which is something we haven't experienced with any other weight loss method. It is a little different for stretch marks; people who think their stretch marks will disappear with this diet will be disappointed. But in terms of elasticity, you have a lot to hope for with HCG. Your skin might not bounce back to the way it was in high school, but it certainly looks better than it would if you lost weight with any other method.

CAUTIONS

There are a few situations in which I would not recommend this weight loss method. One patient of mine had a particular hormone-sensitive breast cancer. While I am not worried that HCG can cause breast cancer—or any cancer, for that matter—her recent survival of this type of cancer was my reason for saying no to her. If she were to use the HCG diet for weight loss and her cancer relapsed for whatever reason later, it would be hard to clear HCG as one of the suspects. Her oncologist agreed, so we explored other options that might work for her. Let me reiterate, I do *not* think HCG can cause cancer; there are no such reports. Rather, we know obesity can cause cancer, as explained in earlier chapters.

Other conditions I have seen in my patients required me to closely monitor their use and progress with the HCG method. Patients with thyroid disease, diabetes, high cholesterol, hypertension, fibromyalgia, arthritis, benign breast lumps, and even brain tumors (prolactinoma) have still been able to use the HCG method, but I have monitored them closely.

The good thing is that HCG does not interact with other medications, so that is not an issue at all. Because of possible low blood sugar, I do adjust insulin and diabetes medicine, and sometimes I decrease blood pressure medicine because a patient's blood pressure improves. But any adjustments I make are not because of medication interaction; they're because the patient experiences improvement of the underlying condition! This is a best-case scenario for doctors and patients.

HOW MY PATIENTS HAVE ADAPTED

The HCG protocol can be difficult to explain to someone who is either unfamiliar with it or critical of it. (Usually, they go hand in hand.) My patients typically tell their families that they are on a "crazy diet" right now. Many just say they are on a low-calorie or low-carb diet. I recently followed up with a patient who shared some of the diet details with a coworker who responded, "How can you survive on that? Just my morning coffee has 500 calories in it!"

I know the HCG diet plan requires patients to make decisions about the foods they eat and activities they partake in. But many people who are able to get their family and friends on board find that they are supportive. One patient informed me that he had gone on vacation with the rest of his family and had to share the details of his diet when they were all eating mahi mahi wrapped in bacon and he was ordering a plain salad with grilled chicken. But they supported him, and he actually stuck to the diet and lost weight on vacation. Now who does that? Rules usually go out the window when you go on vacation! The point is that involving your family and friends in your plans to eat healthfully and adapt your lifestyle can keep you on track—and inspire them to make similar changes.

HCG—WHAT WILL IT TAKE?

What is it going to take for the HCG method of weight loss to become more accepted in the medical community? First, we need to remove all the fake versions of the hormone that are out there. The homeopathic versions containing mere traces of HCG need to go away as well, because they change the data that is available. And those who are prescribing the method need to stick with the original protocol as closely as possible.

Not every doctor has studied and researched this method. I have had patients say that the HCG method did not work for them in a doctor's clinic. I tell them that they cannot fail the HCG method unless they're doing the program incorrectly. Some say they received injections only three times a week. Wrong; it needs to be every day. Others were told to eat 500 calories, but it was not a specified diet. Wrong; the original protocol was very specific. Some were given another shot to help speed up the fat burning process—this is not protocol! It is really up to you to do your research (and I hope this book helps!). Because I researched the diet extensively, I knew what I was getting into and could tell if the program I was considering was real or if the clinic was simply trying to make money.

Insurance does not cover the program, since the FDA believes it is placebo in terms of weight loss uses. I honestly think it's just an excuse for them not to pay—just like they rarely want to pay for any weight loss related procedures.

I have heard of all kinds of different prices for HCG diet programs. When I went to the clinic in Dallas, the six-week protocol cost me $1,500. I was fine with that, because I knew they were administering the method the way they were supposed to, and I also learned some things from them on how to do it right. But I don't want to limit patients who can't afford that amount. In my clinic, I charge only $100 a week ($600 total for the six weeks). Lab work, weekly body composition analysis, the medication, supplies, and access to my staff and me by phone any time of the day, seven days a week, are all included in that price. I also work around their budgets, allowing them to pay over a longer period if they need to. I'm not trying to make money off this. HCG helped me regain my health, and I want to offer the same—health, hope—to my patients.

CHAPTER 11

LIFE AFTER
WEIGHT LOSS

AS you've seen—both in this book and firsthand—one size does *not* fit all when it comes to weight loss. Depending on what has caused your weight gain (and I hope you've been able to figure that out!), certain diets and programs will work better for you than others. One thing, however, is consistent across the board: life after weight loss can be difficult. And it doesn't have to be.

DIET FUSION: CUSTOMIZING YOUR OWN DIET PLAN

Even though I fully endorse HCG as a rapid weight loss method, you need to have a long-term plan. After a patient loses weight—either on HCG or another program—I often recommend what I call "diet fusion." This is when we customize a diet program that I believe will work best for a particular individual based on his or her preferences and ability to make the necessary changes. In order to be successful, you must find something that works for you and your lifestyle.

I start by considering the options from different diets. For one patient, I combined the higher protein from the Atkins diet with the low-carb (not no-carb) portion from the South Beach diet. Then we used the point system from

Weight Watchers to figure out how much she was going to be eating every day. We did this because she had a lot of trouble with carbs and portion control. For another patient, eating every three hours made sense because he worked long hours on the field and couldn't take long breaks for meals while on duty. Then I recommended incorporating aspects of the Richard Simmons program or P90X for exercise. The lesson here? By taking the "best" parts of each of these diets and combining them in a way that is realistic, you are more likely to successfully integrate these healthier habits into your life.

PLAN TO SUCCEED!

As we *all* know, it's easier to gain weight than it is to lose it. We've talked about the science behind this: few fat cells beget more fat cells, whereas weight loss triggers the innate biological processes that oppose permanent weight loss. In other words, the weight *will* come back if you pick up your old habits. Our goal, then, is to keep up the fight and stake our claim to this new and lower set point! The way to do this is by creating a plan to keep the old habits away.

Of course, this is where people often fall short.

I recommend my patients have a written plan for life after weight loss. One of the first things I recommend to my patients for life after weight loss is to have a *written plan*. If you were trying to succeed in business, wouldn't you draft a business plan? Maintaining good health is similar—you need to have a step-by-step action plan that will help you to your next goal, next phase, or a place where you can sustain all your achievements.

As with a business plan, your written goals should be clear, specific, and realistic. Share them—including the timeline in which you want to achieve them—and reward yourself when you reach each one. My first goal after I reached my ideal weight of 180 was simple: *do not regain the lost pounds!*

I decided that as the first step in achieving my goal, I would weigh myself every morning and stick to that same daily routine. I get up, empty my bladder, and stand on the scale. I know that my weight is most stable in the morning, and I keep a log so I can hold myself accountable. Accountability is key. Consider sharing your goal with someone else and reporting back to him or her whether or not you've achieved or maintained it.

Beside each goal, write down a reward that motivates you to accomplish it. One way I have rewarded myself is by putting a quarter in a piggy bank (yup) every day that I remember to weigh myself. Those quarters add up, and I promised to treat myself to a new dress or outfit once it became a substantial sum, say $50. So, every six months, I should have enough in the piggy bank to buy something. (After I got tired of looking for daily quarters, I put dollar bills in the jar instead.) The idea is to reward yourself in a way that motivates you to keep up with the goals you have created for yourself.

My second goal: *do not regain the lost pounds!*

I decided my second means of achieving this was by not eating junk food. I knew which foods I needed to avoid— that delicious Breyer's ice cream or French fries or fried chicken or another favorite of mine: popsicles! I can't eat just one; I have to devour three or four, so I don't buy them anymore. I simply avoid having junk food within reach. My mom often teases me when she opens my refrigerator and all she finds are apples or baby carrots, but I know that if I keep the healthy options in my house, I am more likely to snack on those instead.

How do I reward myself for not eating junk food? It's a little funny—maybe counterintuitive—but on occasional days when I'm out with family and friends and don't have access to other types of foods, I allow myself some of my "forbidden fruits." Maybe I'll have a cup of Breyer's ice cream at my mom's house or some French fries at a theme park. And that's okay, because I limit this "reward" to just once or twice a month when I'm in these situations.

My third goal: *do not regain the lost pounds!*

I decided my third means of achieving this was to maintain my activity level. While I was on the HCG diet, I was doing about 30 to 50 minutes a day of exercise maybe three times a week, and it wasn't bad. Now I do low-impact aerobic exercise, such as the elliptical, for 30 minutes, and then some abs crunches or light weight work for another 20 minutes. I don't have to do more vigorous exercise to keep the weight off because I didn't do vigorous exercise to *get* the weight off.

My reward for maintaining my exercise routine and activity level? Well ... I allow myself to have an occasional popsicle. I still don't go out and buy them, but if I *happen* to find myself at the house of a friend with young children (prime popsicle location!), I might allow myself to have one once a week as long as I keep up with my exercise routine.

Maintaining your weight loss is really about customization and planning. I'm not going to sit here and tell you I follow all my own rules all the time. Of course not! Stuff happens, life happens—but the majority of the time, because I have written my goals down, I stick to them.

THE FEAR OF FAT

After my patients have reached their goal weight, I try to encourage them to get to a point of self-acceptance, where they are not afraid of fat or pounds. I have found that even after reaching their goal weight according to my calculations, some people may still be a few pounds heavier than what *textbooks* say they should be—so now they want to reach the textbook ideal weight. And some patients, even once they reach *that* number, still see themselves as fat or don't like the way they look.

A patient I recently saw had reached negative five percent obesity based on her body composition. (This was obviously not on HCG because on the protocol, you simply stop losing once all excess body fat has been consumed.) Negative five percent obesity means that she now weighed less than she was supposed to weigh for her height. I showed her how, based on her muscle and fat percentages, she was now underweight. She responded by telling me how big her hips still looked and saying she wanted to find a way to reduce their size. She is still spending a lot of time in the gym trying to target those areas, while I'm trying to keep her from going into the anorexic range.

I believe that God has created us in various shapes, colors, sizes, and frames, and you have to realize that you can't compare yourself to a particular person. I am not teaching weight loss skills to get you to look like a maga-zine model; I'm trying to reduce your health risk. In the process of doing that, I pray and hope that I am not turn-ing patients into people who are just afraid of fat, obsessed with a number on the scale; that is not the goal. The goal is for them to be afraid for their health and afraid of the consequences from excess weight but to accept that nor-mal weight is fine, *even* if it is slightly higher than the next person. Normal weight for you might not be normal weight for the someone else, which is why I focus on body composition and recommend you do the same.

There are a lot of tools online that can help calculate most of these numbers by asking you several questions. Dis-covery Health (www.discoveryhealth.com) is one good resource where you can find calculators for things such as your BMR and metabolic age. If you want to calculate your muscle mass, you can turn to a doctor, a personal trainer, or a body composition scale, which you can find online or at stores like Walmart, Bed, Bath & Beyond, and others. If you're in this weight loss journey alone, knowing these numbers can help you understand what *your* ideal weight loss—not someone else's—should be.

LIFETIME HABITS

It's important—and easier than you think—to develop lifetime habits of staying active once you've lost weight. Even though I have given myself a goal of about three hours of exercise per week, I still try to do things that are more active than if I weren't thinking about it. For example, I might take the stairs at work if I'm only going up a few flights. I might walk or ride my bike, or take my lunch break at a local park, where I can get some fresh air and stretch a little. In terms of socializing, I recently decided to go dancing instead of watching a movie, and I was able to burn calories while learning to salsa instead of consuming calories while *eating* salsa!

So pick your daily living activities wisely and in a health conscious way: walk your pet, sweep your sidewalk, mow your own lawn, or do other things around your house that burn additional calories per day. There are a lot of health and fitness apps out there that you can download on your smart phone or computer that can help you track your activities and burned calories per day. (Just search for "health" and/or "fitness" in your app store or online.) As mentioned earlier, I use one called dailyburn. Pedometers are also helpful to keep track of how many steps you are taking each day.

For now, know that you've already taken the *biggest* step—making the effort to know more about your body in order to weigh less and be healthier. By continuing to be proactive, you *will* find success on your weight loss journey. And I would love to hear all about it. Share your story with me or ask questions by sending me an email or visiting my website. I also see patients in my clinic in San Antonio, Texas, for a free consultation.

DrO@knowmoreweighless.com

1200 Brooklyn Ave, Suite 310
San Antonio, TX 78212

210.475.0605

A CAUSE **BIGGER THAN MYSELF**

THERE are over two billion overweight people worldwide. These are people who have gained excess pounds for reasons both simple and complicated. In this book, we have spent time talking about people who struggle to say "no" to food, people whose emotions run deeper than a gallon of Breyers ice cream can cure, people who are desperate to break free from the weight of their own bodies. I was one of these people. I know the struggle. Yet, I try to keep my experience in perspective by reminding myself of one fact: one sixth of all the people in this world live in chronic hunger.

You can call it a tool or life maintenance guide, but when I am thinking I cannot refuse that extra piece of cake, or I can't seem to find the motivation to climb onto my bike, I remember the billion people in the world who are fighting hunger. According to the Food and Agriculture Organization, while 60 percent of Americans are fighting excess weight, one-third of the people in Africa are fighting hunger.

Growing up in Africa, I saw some of this hunger first-hand. Nigeria is a prime example of a country with a great income disparity. As a leading exporter of petroleum oil, the country is home to some *extremely* wealthy individuals—but the majority of citizens are poor. I remember seeing examples of these two populations in school: the *ajebotas,* or "butter-eaters," were the kids whose families lived on an extremely high income, while the *ajepakos,* or "wood-eaters," were those whose families were so poor the kids had nothing to put into their mouths. The extreme difference between these two groups in the same school environment made no sense to me. How could some have so much while others had nothing? With such wealth in the country, there was—is—no need for 60 percent of the population to live below the poverty line.

And this is not only a problem in Africa. Worldwide, the statistics of hunger are devastating. A child under the age of five dies every five seconds from hunger or hunger-related diseases. That's almost nine million children each year! Yet, two billion people in developed nations are having trouble dealing with their excess weight. Does that mean we should feel guilty for what we have? No, but I keep this in mind when comments like, "I'm starving!" want to escape my lips. Am I really starving? No. But I do know what starvation is and what it can do to a body, a mind, and a spirit, and I am empathetic toward people living in those situations. I remind myself that, while I am fighting the urge to pop that extra snack into my mouth, there are millions looking for just a few grains to eat.

There are things we all can do to fight world hunger—and I think we should. First, we can start by saying no to excess and waste. For example, don't put more than you should eat on your plate. If the whole world is not too busy making consumables for the U.S., other countries might start working on feeding their own people. Conserve energy. With a reduced demand for fuel, global commodity prices—which spike as the cost of fuel for shipping rises each year—can remain more stable, and poorer countries can afford more food. We can also donate a certain dollar amount for every pound we successfully lose to a reputable hunger charity. For example, I chose to donate $1 for every pound I lost to an organization called Action Against Hunger. I plan to continue donating, including proceeds from this book, to this organization. Other organizations worth learning about are Freedom From Hunger, Feed the Children, and Food for the Hungry. You can also use your U.S. citizenship to influence the nation's government policies by joining one (or more) U.S. anti-hunger advocacy/public policy organizations or other organizations that deal with key issues affecting poor people; two such organizations are Bread for the World and the Food Research and Action Center. Volunteering at your local food bank or soup kitchen is another way to get involved locally. Please visit my website, www.knowmoreweighless.com, for more information on helping or donating to this cause, as well as for additional tools to empower you on your weight loss journey. You'll be among good company for the ride!

—Dr. O

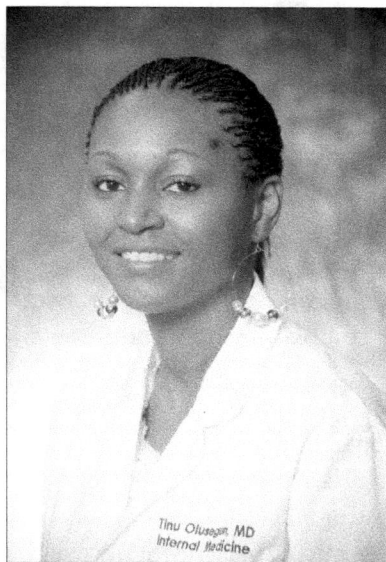

ABOUT
THE
AUTHOR

Growing up in West Africa, Dr. Tinuade Olusegun—"Dr. O" to her patients—experienced healthcare delivery to the underserved and underprivileged first-hand. She vowed, at an early age, to make patient care her life's work and emigrated to the United States to realize that dream.

Dr. O earned her Bachelor of Science degree at the University of Maryland in College Park, Maryland and completed medical school training at Virginia Commonwealth University/Medical College of Virginia. She later obtained post-graduate education in internal medicine, completing her internship and residency at Georgetown University Hospital/Washington Hospital Center in Washington, D.C.

After residency, Dr. O relocated from the northeast U.S. to Texas and began practice as an internal medicine hospitalist at Baylor University Medical Center in downtown Dallas. Dr. O worked with renowned specialists in all fields of medicine, helping her gain even further insight into human diseases. Along the way, she realized that many of the conditions she was treating were secondary to being overweight or obese. Heart disease, diabetes, arthritis, pulmonary difficulty—many times these problems stem from the mysterious disease called obesity. Dr. O knew that if she could just help her patients lose weight, many of their complaints would be automatically addressed.

She has spent the years researching obesity and its causes and treatment, and helping patients develop customized, effective weight loss solutions. *Know More, Weigh Less* synthesizes her knowledge and experience with weight gain and loss, and she hopes it will empower people to understand the disease in order to conquer it—for good.